C0042 17383

D0130421

Heart Health

Your Questions Answered

Glasgow City Council
Cultural & Leisure Services
Libraries Info & Learning
AN

C 004217383

Askews   WITHDRAWN   01-Apr-2009

616.12   FH   £9.99

Heart Health

Your Questions Answered

Dr Robert Ascheim & Dr Deborah Ascheim

Dr Chris Davidson (Consultant)

DK

LONDON, NEW YORK, MUNICH, MELBOURNE, DELHI

Senior Editor Peter Jones
Senior Art Editor Sara Robin
Executive Managing Editor Adèle Hayward
Managing Art Editor Kat Mead
Production Editor Ben Marcus
Production Controller Hema Gohil
Art Director Peter Luff
Publisher Stephanie Jackson

Produced for Dorling Kindersley by
Editor Pip Morgan
Designer Edward Kinsey

Text for Chapters 6 & 7
written by Dr. Penny Preston

This edition first published in the United Kingdom in 2008 by
Dorling Kindersley Limited, 80 Strand, London WC2R 0RL
A Penguin Company

2 4 6 8 10 9 7 5 3 1

Every effort has been made to ensure that the information in this book is accurate.
The information in this book may not be applicable in each individual case so you are therefore
advised to obtain expert medical advice for specific information on personal health matters. Never
disregard expert medical advice or delay in receiving advice or treatment due to information
obtained from this book. The naming of any product, treatment, or organization in this book does
not imply endorsement by the authors, imprimatur, or publisher, nor does the omission of such
names indicate disapproval. The publisher, authors, and imprimatur cannot accept legal
responsibility for any personal injury or other damage or loss arising from any use or misuse
of the information and advice in this book.

Copyright © 2008 Dorling Kindersley Limited, London
Text copyright © 2008 Dr Robert Ascheim and Dr Deborah Ascheim
The authors have asserted their moral right to be identified as the authors of this work.

All rights reserved. No part of this publication may be reproduced, stored in a retrieval system,
or transmitted in any form or by any means, electronic, mechanical, photocopying, recording,
or otherwise, without the prior written permission of the copyright owners.All enquiries
regarding any extracts or reuse of any material in this book should be addressed to
the publishers, Dorling Kindersley Limited.

A CIP catalogue record for this book is available from the British Library.
ISBN: 9781405331111

Printed in China by Hung Hing
Colour reprographics by MDP, England

See our complete catalogue at
www.dk.com

Foreword

The treatment of heart problems has made huge advances in the last 50 years. Pacemakers, heart-lung pumps, almost the entire spectrum of antihypertensive medications, the statin medications, cardiac transplantation, sophisticated cardiac surgery, the understanding and treatment of arrhythmias, the cardiac care unit – all are products of the last half a century.

Our aim in this book is to give you, the reader, the most up-to-date understanding of heart disease and of how it is treated. If we have succeeded, you will know what a heart attack is, how it is different from a stroke, and you will be able to define heart failure. This understanding should translate into behaviour that will stave off these maladies or, if they occur, you will be equipped to understand the rationale behind the treatment.

Dr Robert Ascheim and Dr Deborah Ascheim

Contents

Understanding your heart
Circulation of blood 10
Chambers and valves 14
The heart beat, pulse, and blood
  pressure 18
Heart muscle 27
Changes to the heart in the womb
  and at birth 29

Risk factors
Age, gender, and family 34
Blood pressure changes 36
Cholesterol 38
Lifestyle risks 40
Obesity and diabetes 50

Heart problems
Coronary artery disease 54
Arrhythmias 60
Valve disorders 67
Heart failure 71
Endocarditis 76

Diagnosing heart problems
Measuring blood pressure 80
Devices to assess the heart 82
Coronary angiograms 87
Blood tests 90

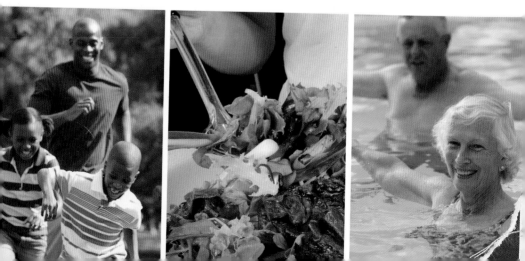

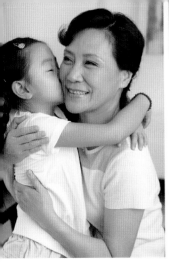
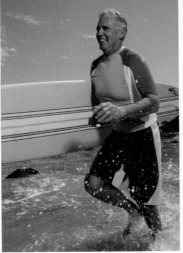
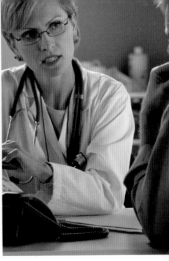

Treating heart disease

Treating acute disorders 94
Treating coronary artery disease 97
Cholesterol-lowering drugs 102
Treating high blood pressure 105
Treating angina 108
Treating arrhythmias 110
Treating heart failure 115
Treating valve disorders 118

Living with coronary artery disease

Recovering from a heart attack 124
The healthy heart lifestyle 132
Finding out your healthy weight 134
A healthy diet 140
Losing weight 147
Reducing cholesterol 148
Salt-restricted diet 150
Giving up smoking 151

Exercise 153
Sex and relationships 157
Coping with stress 158
Dealing with depression 160

Special groups

Heart problems in old age 164
Heart problems in children 166
Heart problems in women 169
Heart problems in diabetics 171
Heart problems and obesity 173

Long-term outlook

Recurring problems 176
Complications 178
Future treatments 181

Useful addresses 184
Index 185
Acknowledgments 192

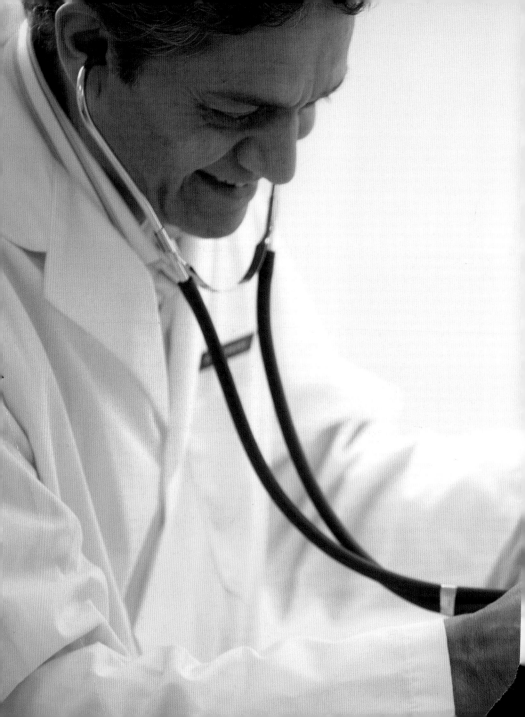

Understanding your heart

Your heart is an extraordinarily reliable and efficient organ that carries on beating more than 2,000 million times in 75 years of life. Sometimes it seems as though you can take it for granted, as if it will carry on regardless, no matter what you do. Understanding its anatomy and how it works will help you to appreciate that looking after your heart is, in fact, essential to your health.

Circulation of the blood

Q Where is my heart exactly?

You probably know where it is because sometimes you can feel it beating. You will find it inside your rib cage, not quite in the centre of your chest, just a little to the left of your breastbone behind the 3rd to the 7th ribs.

Q What does my heart do?

Your heart pumps the total volume of your blood – approximately 5 litres (9 pints) – around your body every minute. In fact, your heart is really two pumps in one that work together. About 70 times a minute the left side pumps blood through your arteries so that every cell in your body receives what it needs to survive and grow (oxygen, glucose, hormones, minerals, vitamins, and other nutrients) and can get rid of its waste products (particularly carbon dioxide). The right side of your heart pumps blood simultaneously to your lungs, where the carbon dioxide is removed and exhaled, and oxygen is absorbed into the blood.

Q Is this circulation all one system?

Yes and no. The two sides of the heart pump blood into two different but connected systems. The main system involves the lion's share of the blood and circulates it around the body. It is called the systemic circulation. The blood going to and from the lungs is transported in the pulmonary circulation (the word pulmonary comes from the Greek and relates to the lung). This is a much shorter system because the lungs are located beside your heart. Taken together these two components of the system – including the heart – are referred to as thecardiovascular system (see p13).

Q What does cardiovascular mean?

Cardiovascular comes from two terms. "Cardio" refers to the heart and "vascular" refers to the blood vessels. Whenever you see or read words such as "cardiac" or "cardiology" you can assume they refer to the heart.

Q What happens in the systemic circulation?

After the blood leaves the heart it flows through various branching blood vessels – arteries, arterioles, capillaries, venules, and veins – until it returns to the heart (see p13). At first, the blood travels along the main arteries until it reaches the tissues, such as the brain, liver, kidneys, and other organs, as well as muscles, nerves, and bones. The blood vessels branch into smaller and smaller vessels known as arterioles, which eventually become tiny capillaries, with walls that are one cell thick. Here the blood delivers nutrients to the cells and picks up waste products. The blood then moves into tiny veins and then larger veins as the circulation returns to the heart.

Q How extensive is the network?

If you put all the body's arteries, arterioles, capillaries, venules, and veins together in a long line they would stretch around the world almost four times. And around 98 per cent of the systemic circulation is composed of an enormous network of capillaries.

Q What is an artery made of?

Arteries are hollow tubes with thick walls that have an outer protective layer, a layer of muscle, an elastic layer, and an inner lining. These layers have to withstand the high-pressure force of the blood as it is pumped out of the heart – a force so strong that a cut artery can spurt blood for several feet. As the wave of pressure passes through, the artery walls expand, then contract.

Q Do veins also have thick walls?

No. The walls of the veins have an outer layer, a muscle layer, and an inner lining. However, they are relatively thin because, unlike the arteries, they do not need to withstand the full force of the heart pumping the blood. In fact, the pressure of the blood in your veins is about one tenth of the pressure in your arteries.

Q Do veins have valves?

Yes. Large veins, such as those in the thigh, have valves that allow blood to flow towards the heart but prevent it from flowing in the other direction and pooling in the feet. Veins can collect a large volume of blood.

Q Where is most of my blood when I am resting?

When your body is resting your veins hold most of your blood (about 70 per cent). The remainder is in your arteries (10 per cent), your lungs (10 per cent), your heart (5 per cent), and in your capillaries (5 per cent).

Q If the pressure in the veins is low, what makes the blood return to the heart?

The main factor that makes the veins carry blood back towards the heart is the muscle pump. The muscles, for instance in the legs, that surround a vein act like a pump as they alternately contract and relax around the stretches of vein. As they contract they squeeze the blood onward against the force of gravity and as they relax, the vein refills with more blood. So it is best for your circulation to remain active.

Q Are there any other factors?

Yes. Gravity in the upper body also encourages the return of blood to the heart. In addition, when you inhale, your rib cage expands and the pressure in your chest falls below the pressure in the rest of your body making blood flow along the veins, towards the chest and the heart.

THE CARDIOVASCULAR SYSTEM

The heart lies at the centre of a very intricate network of blood vessels called the cardiovascular system. In a continuous cycle, the heart receives oxygenated blood (red) from the lungs and pumps it into the arteries. It then receives deoxygenated blood (blue) returning from the body via the veins and pumps it into the lungs.

This illustration shows the major blood vessels in the cardiovascular system. The red arterial network is shown on the right side of the body (left side of the picture) and the blue venous network on the left. In reality, both sides of the body are similarly supplied. The heart pumps blood into the aorta, which has branches to the head, the arms, the major organs, and to all parts of the body. Returning to the heart, veins eventually channel blood into two major veins – the superior vena cava (SVC) brings blood from the upper half of the body, while the inferior vena cava (IVC) collects blood from the lower half of the body.

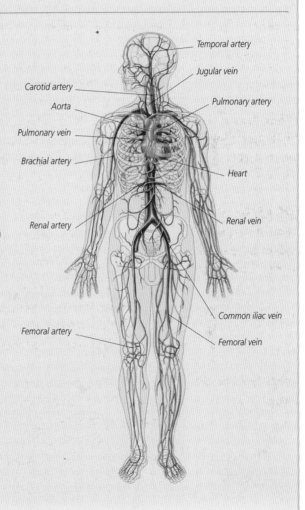

Temporal artery

Jugular vein

Carotid artery

Pulmonary artery

Aorta

Pulmonary vein

Brachial artery

Heart

Renal artery

Renal vein

Common iliac vein

Femoral artery

Femoral vein

Chambers and valves

Q How big is my heart?

Your heart is about the size of a clenched fist – about 12.5cm (5in) long, 7.5cm (3in) thick, and 8.75cm (3.5in) across at its widest, although a heart can grow in size, especially in males, for many years. If you are a woman your heart probably weighs 225g to 280g (8–10oz), while for men the heart is a little heavier, weighing between 280g and 340g (10–12oz).

Q What are the component parts of the heart?

The heart is a hollow, muscular pump with two halves. The right and left half each have two chambers and two sets of valves. These two distinct halves are completely separated by a thick wall, or septum. Each half has an upper chamber called an atrium (it used to be called an auricle) and a lower chamber called a ventricle (see p16).

Q What does the right half of the heart do?

The right atrium of the heart receives oxygen-poor blood from two large veins – the superior vena cava and the inferior vena cava. As it contracts it moves the blood through the tricuspid valve into the right ventricle. The right ventricle pumps this blood, which is dark purple in colour, through the pulmonary valve into the pulmonary artery and then on to the lungs.

Q What does the left half of the heart do?

The left atrium of the heart receives freshly oxygenated blood from the lungs via the pulmonary vein and then pushes it through the mitral valve into the left ventricle. The left ventricle then pumps the oxygen-rich blood, which is pink-orange in colour, through the aortic valve into the aorta and then around the body.

THE STRUCTURE OF THE HEART

The heart is conical in shape, with its apex pointing downward, slightly forward and to the left. It is composed largely of muscle and is an extraordinarily efficient pump. It has four chambers, of which the upper two – the atria – are receiving chambers and the bottom two – the ventricles – are the pumping chambers.

The ventricular chambers are formed by muscle known as the myocardium, which is three times thicker on the left side than on the right to cope with the higher pressures. The heart is in a sac called the pericardium, which is anchored to the surrounding tissues. The chambers contract and relax in a regular sequence called the cardiac cycle (see pp18–23) and blood consequently flows through the four valves along pressure gradients. The right atrium receives blood from the superior vena cava and the inferior vena cava, and the left atrium receives blood from the lungs via the pulmonary veins. The right ventricle pumps blood into the pulmonary artery and the left ventricle pumps blood into the aorta.

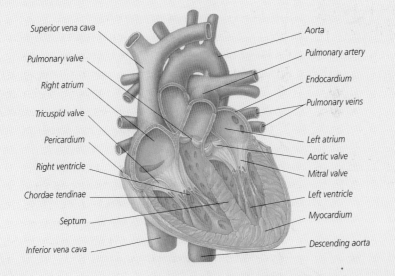

Superior vena cava
Pulmonary valve
Right atrium
Tricuspid valve
Pericardium
Right ventricle
Chordae tendinae
Septum
Inferior vena cava

Aorta
Pulmonary artery
Endocardium
Pulmonary veins
Left atrium
Aortic valve
Mitral valve
Left ventricle
Myocardium
Descending aorta

Q Don't veins carry deoxygenated blood?

Everywhere else in the body the veins carry deoxygenated blood, but the convention is that vessels bringing blood *to* the heart are called veins whereas vessels that take blood *away* from the heart are called arteries. So the vessel taking deoxygenated blood from the right ventricle of the heart to the lungs is an artery and the blood vessels bringing oxygenated blood from the lungs to the left atrium of the heart are veins.

Q Are the ventricles the same size?

No. The left ventricle is bigger because it is the major pumping chamber in the heart and has to pump blood at higher pressures to adequately circulate to the whole body. It is on average about three times the thickness of the right ventricle.

Q Does this mean that the left ventricle pumps more blood than the right?

No. It's important that both ventricles have the same output per minute. If they are unequal, as in the case of heart failure when at least one of the ventricles is weak, then blood circulation becomes ineffective.

Q What are the valves made of?

There are four valves inside the heart that control the flow of blood into and out of the ventricles. They have cup-shaped flaps, cusps, that are made predominantly of a tough protein called collagen to cope with the pressure. The tricuspid, pulmonary, and aortic valves have three cusps and the mitral valve has two.

Q How are the valves held in place?

Each cusp in the larger mitral and tricuspid valves is tethered to the wall of the heart by tough fibrous strands called chordae tendinae. As these valves open and close these strands prevent the pressure and flow of the blood from turning the cusp inside out.

Q How do the valves work?

Valves enable the blood to flow in only one direction. Basically, the pressure difference of the blood in adjacent chambers opens and closes the cusps of a valve. For example, when the right atrium contracts the pressure of the blood inside becomes higher than the blood in the right ventricle, so the tricuspid valve opens, allowing blood through. When the pressure in the right ventricle rises, the tricuspid valve closes, so that the blood flows only in the forward direction.

Q Why can you hear the heart beat?

If you listen to someone's heart with a stethoscope you will hear the sounds of the heart as it goes through its pumping cycle (see pp18–23). It seems like a soft voice repeatedly saying "lub-dup". The first heart sound, the "lub", is the sound of the mitral and tricuspid valves closing. The second heart sound, the "dup", is the sound of the pulmonary and aortic valves closing. After the "dup" there is a slight pause before the next "lub".

Q What holds the heart in position?

The heart and base of the large vessels that enter and leave the heart are held in the pericardium. This big, double-layered membrane allows the heart to move without friction in the chest. It is anchored to the diaphragm below the heart, to the breastbone in front of the heart, and to connective tissue behind the heart.

Q Does the heart have a lining?

Yes. A smooth membrane, the endocardium, lines the internal surfaces to keep blood from sticking. It is continuous with the lining of the vessels, such as the aorta, that enter and leave the heart. It is thicker in the atria than the ventricles and thickest of all in the left atrium.

The heartbeat, pulse, and blood pressure

Q What is the heartbeat?

Your heart beats once for each complete sequence of the cardiac cycle – receiving blood from the veins, then pumping it to the lungs, receiving it from the lungs, then pumping it into the aorta (see pp20–21). You can hear it as the heart sounds (see p17).

Q Is the pulse my doctor "feels" the same as my heartbeat?

Not quite but they are related. When the heart beats and the blood is pumped into the aorta, a pressure wave spreads along the arteries of the body at about 6m (20ft) per second and expands the arterial walls. You can feel this wave as the pulse in places where an artery comes close to the skin – for example, where the radial artery passes through the wrist.

Q What are doctors doing when they "feel" my pulse?

They are determining your heart rate by counting the number of pressure waves per minute. This tells them how many cardiac cycles your heart completes in a minute. It is one sign of the health of your heart.

Q Are there any other places where doctors can "feel" the pulse?

Yes, in several places: in the crook of the arm where the brachial artery passes above the elbow; in the femoral artery at the top of the thigh between the groin and hip; and in the carotid artery in the neck just below the jaw. The femoral pulse is often felt during cardiac resuscitation (see p95) because it is one of the last pulses to disappear and the first to reappear.

Q How often does the heart beat?

The heart of a healthy adult who is resting beats between 60 and 80 times per minute. The heart rate speeds up considerably during activity, whether it is walking, gardening, cycling, or playing some sort of sport. During strenuous exercise it can beat as many as 200 times a minute. This speeding up occurs because the cells of the body's tissues, particularly the muscles, need plenty of oxygen and glucose delivered rapidly so that they can generate energy. In addition, they need the blood to quickly remove the toxic waste products of their metabolism.

Q Does the heart beat when its muscle contracts?

Basically, the cardiac cycle has three phases. During the first phase, called diastole (pronounced *dy-as-tollee*), the heart's muscles relax and blood flows into the atria and ventricles. During the second phase, called atrial systole (pronounced *sis-tollee*), the muscles of the two atria contract, pumping the remaining atrial blood into the ventricles. During the third phase, called ventricular systole, the valves between the atria and the ventricles close, and the muscles of the two ventricles contract, pumping the blood out of the heart. (See pp20–21.)

Q How is the heartbeat started?

Essentially there is a sophisticated electrical system in the heart that includes a pacemaker (see p20), which sends out electrical signals timed to the cardiac cycle. Its signals are conducted along specialized muscle fibres that function like electrical wires and trigger the second phase of the cycle by making the muscles of the atria contract. The vagus nerve brings impulses from the brain and controls the minute-by-minute changes to the heart rate.

How the heart beats

The movement of the blood through the four chambers of the heart is one example of the body's extraordinary feats of timing. The beating of the healthy heart is an all-or-nothing process that involves every cardiac muscle cell contracting and relaxing in time to the carefully controlled electrical rhythm of the tiny pacemaker. This sinoatrial node is like an unflappable conductor synchronizing the various instruments of a large orchestra. The heart cycle is a pattern that repeats itself more than 100,000 times each day, as valves open and close, and the heart fills with blood and then pumps it out again.

THE HEART'S PACEMAKER

The heart's pacemaker, the sinoatrial node, is embedded in the wall of the right atrium, close to where the superior vena cava brings venous blood from the upper part of the body. The sinoatrial node contains specialized cardiac cells that initiate the wave of electricity which triggers the heart muscles to contract.

First, it makes the muscles of the atria contract—the first part of the heartbeat. Then, after a split-second delay, it stimulates the atrioventricular node, located on the opposite side of the right atrium, to boost the wave of electricity and send it down either side of the wall separating the two ventricles. It spreads out and coordinates the contraction of the muscle cells in both ventricles.

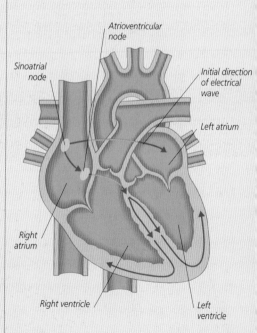

Atrioventricular node

Sinoatrial node

Initial direction of electrical wave

Left atrium

Right atrium

Right ventricle

Left ventricle

THE HEART CYCLE

The heart cycle, also called the cardiac cycle, is the repeating pattern of relaxation (diastole) and contraction (systole) that the pacemaker coordinates as it controls the passage of blood through the chambers of the heart.

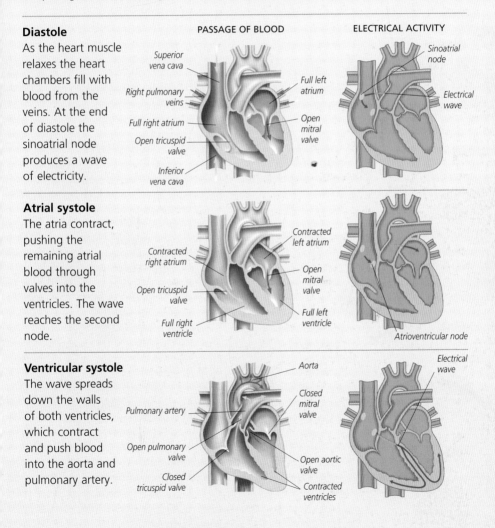

PASSAGE OF BLOOD   ELECTRICAL ACTIVITY

Diastole

As the heart muscle relaxes the heart chambers fill with blood from the veins. At the end of diastole the sinoatrial node produces a wave of electricity.

Superior vena cava
Right pulmonary veins
Full right atrium
Open tricuspid valve
Inferior vena cava
Full left atrium
Open mitral valve
Sinoatrial node
Electrical wave

Atrial systole

The atria contract, pushing the remaining atrial blood through valves into the ventricles. The wave reaches the second node.

Contracted right atrium
Open tricuspid valve
Full right ventricle
Contracted left atrium
Open mitral valve
Full left ventricle
Atrioventricular node

Ventricular systole

The wave spreads down the walls of both ventricles, which contract and push blood into the aorta and pulmonary artery.

Pulmonary artery
Open pulmonary valve
Closed tricuspid valve
Aorta
Closed mitral valve
Open aortic valve
Contracted ventricles
Electrical wave

Q **What makes the ventricles contract?**

The signals from the pacemaker reach another node, called the atrioventricular node, in the muscle wall near the bottom left of the right atrium (see p21). This second node sends a wave of electrical signals through the walls of both ventricles, causing them to contract in the third phase of the cardiac cycle.

Q **What does adrenaline do to my heart rate?**

Whenever you are afraid, or get excited, emotional, or angry, your adrenal glands release adrenaline and other hormones into your bloodstream. This fast-acting hormone increases your heart rate – your heart feels like it's pounding – so that more blood goes to your muscles and brain, and less to your stomach and skin. If you have a shock or lose a significant amount of blood, adrenaline will raise your blood pressure.

Q **What is blood pressure?**

When the heart pumps blood into the aorta it generates a pressure wave that spreads along the arteries, causing them to expand. This blood pressure is precisely linked to the phases of the cardiac cycle (see pp20–21) and is the difference between the pressure when the heart beats (systole) and when it relaxes (diastole).

Q **Is this why there are always two readings when my blood pressure is tested?**

Yes. For a normal healthy adult the two readings are 120 (at systole) and 80 (at diastole), meaning the blood pressure is 120 over 80, or 120/80 for short. Before digital machines, the blood pressure was measured by seeing how far it could push up a column of mercury. Doctors and medical scientists still use this measure, though the method of obtaining it has changed. Hence, normal systolic pressure is 120mm of mercury (Hg, for short) and normal diastolic pressure is 80mm mercury.

Q Is the blood pressure the same in the pulmonary circulation?

No, the pulmonary circulation is a relatively low-pressure system compared to the systemic circulation. It is not often measured and then only with a cardiac catheter, a tube inserted into the heart. The blood pressure in the pulmonary artery during the cardiac cycle, for example, ranges between 25 and 10mm of mercury, so the pulmonary artery pressure is 25/10mm of mercury.

BLOOD SUPPLY TO THE HEART

The vitally important cells in your heart muscle are supplied with blood via the two main coronary arteries. They are the first arteries to branch off the aorta and they receive around five per cent of the blood that the heart pumps out. Their name comes from the way they cover both sides of the heart like a crown (*corona* is Latin for crown).

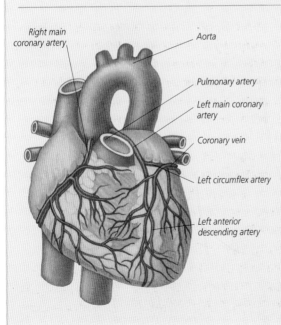

Right main coronary artery

Aorta

Pulmonary artery

Left main coronary artery

Coronary vein

Left circumflex artery

Left anterior descending artery

The coronary arteries are like arteries in every way, except for the fact that blood primarily flows through them during diastole, when the heart relaxes. This means that the cells of the heart muscle receive their supply of blood and have their waste products removed *after* they have contracted and *before* they contract again. The coronary veins return blood to the heart via the right atrium.

Q How is blood pressure controlled?

Keeping blood pressure under control is very important. If it is too low, not enough blood gets to the cells of the body and tissues are damaged, but if it's too high the blood vessels and tissues are damaged as well.Controlling blood pressure involves a number of different bodily mechanisms. Changes of blood pressure in the short term – for example, when you suddenly stand from a sitting position – are quickly corrected by centres in the brain and nervous system, which adjust the heart rate and the diameter of the arteries. Hormones control blood pressure in the long term by adjusting the contraction of the arteries and volume of fluid excreted by the kidneys, which regulates the volume of blood and consequently its pressure.

Q How do the arteries and arterioles of the body change in diameter?

The walls of these blood vessels contain a layer of muscle that can relax and contract. You cannot voluntarily control this kind of muscle (called smooth muscle), but it is controlled by the nervous system. When the nervous system stimulates the muscles to contract, the diameters of the arteries and arterioles get smaller. This constriction narrows the blood vessels, thereby causing the blood pressure to increase. When the muscles are "told" to relax, these blood vessels widen (known as dilation) and the blood pressure falls.

Q How do the arteries help control blood pressure?

In the carotid arteries in the neck, as well as inside the heart, stretch receptors called baroreceptors ("baro" refers to pressure as in a barometer) are sensitive to changes in blood pressure. When these cells detect a rise in pressure they trigger the nervous system to widen the arterioles in the body so that the blood pressure drops.

Q If I give a pint of blood, does my blood pressure change?

Yes, your blood pressure falls, which can make you light-headed. The cardiovascular system compensates by increasing the heart rate and then constricting the blood vessels, thereby normalizing the blood pressure. This process takes a few minutes, which is why you rest, generally lying down, after giving blood.

Q Does gravity have an effect on blood pressure?

Yes. When you stand upright, blood tends to pool in the lower half of your body. Blood pressure rises below the heart but decreases above it. As a general rule, blood pressure changes by about 10mm of mercury for every 12cm (5in) from the heart. So if the normal systolic pressure is 120mm of mercury at the aorta, it will be about 210mm at the feet and only 90mm in the brain. When you lie down, these pressures will be 120mm.

Q Does blood pressure increase with age?

Yes. It's quite natural and the increase is not very significant in normal circumstances. As you grow older the walls of your arteries and arterioles thicken, so they become narrower. The walls also become less elastic, so the smooth muscle in the walls cannot relax or contract as easily or as effectively. As a result, they are less effective at controlling blood pressure (see p24).

Q Does my blood pressure vary throughout the 24-hour day?

Yes. Your blood pressure falls while you are asleep, perhaps between 10mm and 20mm of mercury. Then, when you wake and stand up, it increases quickly. Usually the highest blood pressure during the day is between 6am and midday. Obviously it depends on what you do during the day, but as a general rule your blood pressure is probably higher while you are working than while you are relaxing.

Myth "Only men have heart attacks"

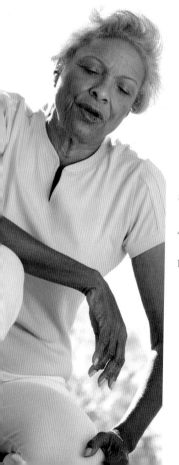

Truth In the past heart attacks have commonly been associated with men, but nothing could be further from the truth. In fact, coronary artery disease is the main cause of death in women above the age of 50, and is second only to cancer for all women. As a general rule, the risk increases after the menopause.

Heart muscle

Q What do heart muscle cells look like?

Heart muscle, often called cardiac muscle, is one of three types of muscle in the body. The other two are skeletal muscle and smooth muscle. Heart muscle is unique and found nowhere else in the body. Looking at heart muscle under the microscope, lots of striations can be seen. These are deep, red fibres, or filaments. Each of the fibres forms branches that come into close contact with the fibres from other heart muscle cells, enabling them to work together as a network.

Q How do the cells work?

Each of the heart muscle cells can contract and relax on its own because it has a kind of rhythmic power. The cells are not directly connected to the nervous system like other types of muscle, but are triggered to contract together by a wave of electricity that is generated by the sinoatrial and atrioventricular nodes (see pp20–21). Nerves can alter the rate and strength of contraction but they don't make the heart beat.

Q Does one cell pass on the electrical signal to the next?

Yes. Heart muscle cells excite one another. When one heart muscle cell – for example, in the right atrium – contracts, it conducts the message to contract to all the other cells around it, so a rapid wave of contraction continues to all parts of the muscle in the right atrium. The message also reaches the muscle cells in the left atrium so that chamber contracts at the same time. But the message does not pass to the ventricles because they are separated from the atria by a septum, so the wave of contraction in the atria dies away.

Q How does the wave of electricity reach the ventricles if the septum is in the way?

The only way is through the atrioventricular node, which is connected to the septum that separates the two ventricles via a bundle of specially modified heart cells. These bundles conduct the wave of contraction down either side of the septum where the wave spreads out and stimulates both ventricles simultaneously.

Q What do contractions look like?

Anyone who has watched an operation on a heart will have seen the way it beats. A contracting heart muscle cell seems to twitch briefly – it never contracts for more than a split second. It shortens, thickens, and then relaxes. The atria contract, pushing blood down into the ventricles, then there's the briefest pause before the ventricles contract. They seem to convulse upward as the muscles squeeze out the blood.

Q How does heart muscle keep going 24 hours a day?

Every cell generates its own energy in tiny powerhouses called mitochondria, which consume oxygen and burn glucose to create the fuel the cell needs for its activities. The muscle cells of the heart need to contract and relax continuously without stopping, so they have larger mitochondria than normal and many more of them. In fact, around 25 per cent of a heart muscle cell may be taken up with mitochondria, and most of the rest with the fibres that contract and relax.

Q Do heart muscle cells need a lot of oxygen?

Yes they do, because of their high energy needs. They absorb oxygen from the blood in the coronary arteries. Most cells only absorb about 30 per cent of the oxygen available in the blood that supplies them. However, heart muscle cells are highly efficient and can absorb as much as 90 per cent of the available oxygen.

Change of heart – in the womb and at birth

Q My husband and I have just conceived our first child. When does its blood begin to circulate?

During the third week of pregnancy your baby will have some rudimentary blood vessels attached to those in the umbilical cord. A simple, tube-like heart will grow in the succeeding days and a complex network of blood vessels will develop. By the fifth week, your baby's basic circulation will be operating – the heart pumps blood through the dorsal aorta and other arteries, then blood returns to the heart via veins. However, your baby will still rely on your placenta and the umbilical cord for all its oxygen and nutrition, and to remove all its waste products, such as carbon dioxide and urea.

Q When does our baby's heart really start beating?

By the sixth week after conception your baby's heart is beating steadily and, by the tenth week, it is beating about 80 times each minute. From about the 28th week a doctor should be able to hear your baby's heartbeat with a foetal stethoscope, which is a trumpet-shaped device. Eventually its heartbeat will fluctuate between 120 and 160 beats a minute. The rate will be a good indication of your baby's well-being.

Q How big is our baby's heart?

It's tiny really, but during the second month in the womb it is large compared to the length of its body – this heart size to body ratio is about 1 to 50 – whereas at birth the proportions are 1 to 120. In an adult the ratio is about 1 to 160.

Q While in my womb how does our baby's heart differ?

Your baby's lungs aren't working yet and the big difference in the heart is a hole, called the foramen ovale. It is between the right and left atria, and enables blood returning from the body to go to the left side as well as the right side of the heart. Because your baby receives its oxygen and removes its carbon dioxide via the umbilical cord and your placenta, its heart doesn't need to pump much blood into the lungs, so the right ventricle shares the pumping duties equally with the left ventricle.

Q Does our baby's circulation have special features in the womb?

Yes. Most of the oxygenated blood from the placenta bypasses the liver via the ductus venosus and empties directly into the right side of the heart via the inferior vena cava. Some blood flows directly from the bottom of the pulmonary artery into the aorta via a short tube called the ductus arteriosus. Your baby's heart then sends deoxygenated blood back to the placenta via the umbilical arteries and receives blood full of oxygen and nutrients via the umbilical vein.

Q How does our baby's heart develop?

As it develops, your baby's heart goes through various remarkable stages. At first it is a fast-growing tube, and then it develops into two chambers – the primitive atria and single ventricle – to improve its ability to pump the blood around the body. Initially, the atria are larger than the ventricles. The single ventricle gradually develops a septum that divides it into two and eventually separates. Before birth your baby's ventricles will have grown larger than the atria and the wall of the left ventricle much thicker than the other cardiac chambers.

Q Is it really true that the development of the human heart resembles other animals' hearts?

To a certain extent. Some have suggested the resemblances mirror some stages in animal evolution. For example, the initial tube-like stage looks a bit like a fish heart. When the baby's heart develops two atria, it bears some similarities to a frog heart. When there are three chambers – two atria and a ventricle – the heart is not unlike that of a turtle or snake. Only when the baby's heart has four chambers is it truly mammalian.

Q Will the contractions during labour affect our baby's heart?

Labour contractions push your baby's head into your pelvis which initially may prompt the heart rate to fall, but the rate rapidly returns to normal. Problems during delivery can be reflected in your baby's heart rate, which will be monitored as a precaution.

Q What will happen to our baby's heart at birth?

From the moment your baby takes its first breath and cries, its circulation changes. The lungs oxygenate the blood and the umbilical circulation ceases to function. As the right ventricle pumps blood to the lungs via the pulmonary artery, the foramen ovale (see p30) starts to shut and will close entirely by the tenth day. At birth, the newborn baby's heart rate falls from about 150 to about 100 beats a minute.

Q What happens to the other vessels that our baby needed in the womb?

The ductus arteriosus, the connection between the pulmonary artery and aorta, contracts and closes between the fourth and tenth days. As the circulation to the placenta ceases to function, the ductus venosus – the vessel that allowed the oxygenated umbilical vein blood to empty directly into the inferior vena cava – closes between the second and fifth days after birth. The umbilical vein becomes a fibrous cord.

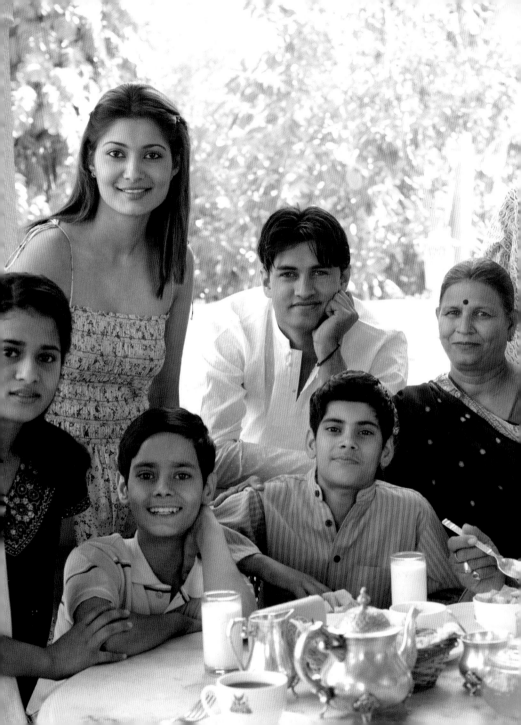

Risk factors

Changes in our lifestyle during the 20th century, combined with the fact that we are living longer, have gone hand in hand with an increase in heart problems. Less exercise, more unhealthy food, increases in the number of people smoking, and elevated levels of stress are all key risk factors, and all those who lead an unhealthy lifestyle endanger the health of their heart.

Age, gender, and family

Q Is a woman of 30 years more, or less, at risk of heart disease than a man of the same age?

You are less at risk. It has often been stated that men develop a disproportionate rate of heart attacks when compared to women. That is so, but only until you reach the age of menopause (see p169). Following menopause, the rate of heart attacks becomes approximately equal in both men and women.

Q Are older people more at risk of heart disease?

Coronary artery disease is a degenerative disease and characteristically is more likely to occur with age. In general, the arteries become less elastic as you grow older so you become more prone to high blood pressure and heart disease. We all know of someone who died suddenly in their 40s, but in general the heart attack is a disease of people over 65.

Q Are there any exceptions?

Of course, there are exceptions, and heart attacks can occur at any age. At one end of the spectrum there are a very small number of people who suffer heart attacks in their 20s. Individuals in this group average a total blood serum cholesterol level in excess of 26 mmol/l (see p38), which is an astonishingly high figure, and rarely survive beyond 30 years of age.

Q Will this risk increase the more elderly I become?

Yes, and the risk is greater for men than women. UK statistics, which are reflected throughout most of Western Europe, show that one in 35 people aged between 65 and 74 develops heart failure (see pp71–75). The chances increase to one in 15 in people between 75 and 84, and to one in seven in people above 85.

Q My parents both died of a heart attack. Am I likely to die of one, too?

You are probably more at risk than someone whose parents did not die of a heart attack. If you have a close relative who died of a heart attack before they were 60 you are more at risk. High cholesterol and high blood pressure are also factors that contribute to your risk of having a heart attack and both can also run in families. You should have these checked from time to time.

Q As a man of south Asian descent, how likely am I to develop cardiovascular disease?

Statistics show that you are more likely than most people in the UK to suffer from fatal heart disease – almost 50 per cent more likely, in fact. Women who are of south Asian descent are similarly at risk. This likelihood is almost certainly linked to your increased risk of developing diabetes.

Q As a woman of Afro-Caribbean descent, is it true that I am less likely to develop heart failure?

Yes, it's true. Statistics show that you are between 25 and 50 per cent less likely to die from heart disease than the average population in the UK. However, evidence also indicates that you are more prone to develop high blood pressure and to experience a stroke.

Q Is there such a thing as a heart attack gene?

No, although many people thought medical scientists engaged in the Human Genome Project – the scheme that mapped human DNA – would discover one. If they had, gene therapy could be targeted to alter that gene and make those who were identified as prone to heart attack less likely to experience this sometimes fatal disease. But the genetic abnormalities involve only a fraction of a gene and involve thousands of different genes. Once the complexities of this "brave new world" are understood, tailored gene therapy to prevent heart attacks may be possible.

Blood pressure changes

Q What is an acceptable blood pressure?

For many decades, 140/90 was considered to be an acceptable blood pressure, but this is no longer so. Community-based studies have demonstrated that people with an average blood pressure of 130/80 have fewer cardiovascular events, so this is now considered to be the accepted optimum blood pressure.

Q Are old people at risk of high blood pressure?

Yes. As people advance in age, their systolic blood pressure increases. This is so common that a "normal" systolic blood pressure was historically considered to be 120 plus one's age. Community-based studies have since shown that older people with an average systolic blood pressure under 130 fared much better than those with higher systolic blood pressure.

Q What are the risks of high blood pressure?

High blood pressure, commonly known as hypertension, does not typically lead to symptoms unless the blood pressure is severely elevated. The most common symptoms include headaches, dizziness, and occasionally blurred vision. Hypertension is often referred to, however, as "the silent killer" because it causes other illnesses (see opposite page) in the absence of symptoms. Untreated hypertension can cause cardiovascular disease in one in three people.

Q Can hypertension cause strokes?

Yes. Strokes, in fact, are the predominant illness caused by high blood pressure. Approximately two in three people who have a stroke also have high blood pressure. This applies to almost twice as many women as men.

Q Is low blood pressure dangerous?

It can be if you're ill. The condition, called shock or hypotension, results in decreased tissue perfusion (not enough blood reaches the tissues). Symptoms depend on which organ is deprived of blood. If it's the brain, light-headedness is the first sign and this can progress all the way to coma. If it's the kidney, less urine is produced and kidney failure can result.

Q What causes low blood pressure?

There are many causes. Common among them are heart attacks which if large enough, result in a heart that cannot pump effectively. Another is the invasion of the blood by certain bacteria that produce a toxin that leads to low blood pressure and inadequate tissue perfusion.

THE PERILS OF HIGH BLOOD PRESSURE

Most people with high blood pressure (hypertension) are either not treated successfully or are not treated at all. Left untreated, high blood pressure can lead to a whole host of problems, including the following:

- Strokes
- Coronary artery disease (If you have hypertension your risk increases between two and three times.)
- Heart attacks
- Congestive heart failure
- Kidney disease
- Hardening of the arteries in the legs (known as peripheral vascular disease)
- Damage to retinal blood vessels (right)

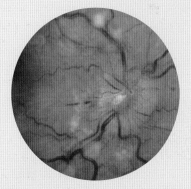

DAMAGE TO RETINAL BLOOD VESSELS

Cholesterol

Q How long have we known about the bad effects of cholesterol?

In the 1850s, a German pathologist named Rudolf Virchow discovered that plaques (atheromata) lining the walls of arteries were composed mostly of cholesterol. Since then it was thought that reducing cholesterol in the blood would reduce the development of atheromata and also lower the incidence of cardiovascular disease. We now know this is true.

Q Cholesterol never used to be such a big problem. Have the risks changed?

When cholesterol became a byword in the 1950s, it was felt that a person would be disadvantaged if their total cholesterol was in excess of 7.75 mmol/l (a mmol stands for millimoles, in which a mole is 6.23×10^{23} molecules). The rules have become progressively more stringent. In the 1960s and 1970s, 6.5 mmol/l became the acceptable upper limit. In the 1980s, this figure was lowered to 6 mmol/l and in the 1990s, below 5 mmol/l became the desired value.

Q I've heard that cholesterol can be good and bad. How is this possible?

In the body, cholesterol circulates with lipoproteins, which are molecules of protein and fat. Two lipoproteins are dominant – high density lipoprotein (HDL) and low density lipoprotein (LDL). They bind with cholesterol and transport it within plasma (a liquid portion of the blood). Medical scientists have discovered that the LDL component traverses the plasma and deposits the cholesterol as atheromata (see p56) on the arterial walls. This is why it is called bad cholesterol. The HDL (good) component acts conversely because it binds with cholesterol and takes it away from the atheromata.

Q So the less LDL I have the lower my risk of coronary artery disease?

Yes. In fact, your LDL cholesterol can't be too low. Ideally, you need a low level of LDL cholesterol and a high level of HDL cholesterol. Formerly, it was thought that a high level of HDL offered protection against a high level of LDL. But this is not the case. An elevated LDL is an independent risk factor for the development of cardiovascular disease. Initially, a level of 3.4 mmol/l was an acceptable LDL level. With more and better studies this was lowered to 2.5 mmol/l. Now, a level of 1.8 mmol/l is considered the optimum.

Q Are there other markers in the blood that indicate a risk of heart disease?

Yes. One is called C Reactive Protein (CRP), which is present when inflammation develops – for example, when plaques (atheromata) form in the lining of arteries and later rupture. CRP may even be directly involved in the disease process. Another is high levels of homocysteine, which is an amino acid.

YOUR CHOLESTEROL RISK

If you are 20 years or older, and don't have diabetes or heart disease, tests can reveal your risk of a heart attack within the foreseeable future by measuring two important cholesterol levels in your blood – total cholesterol and HDL (good) cholesterol.

TOTAL CHOLESTEROL LEVEL
Less than 5 mmol/l (mmol/l stands for millimoles per litre) is the desirable level. Between 5 and 6 mmol/l is borderline, but still a risk. If you have a level of 6 mmol/l or above you are definitely at risk of heart disease.

HDL CHOLESTEROL LEVEL
A level of 1.5 mmol/l and above is healthy and should even protect you from heart disease. A level between 1.5 and 1 mmol/l is borderline. But if the level falls below 1 mmol/l you are at risk from heart disease.

Lifestyle risks

Q My husband is a bit of a couch potato – is he at risk of heart disease?

If he's a couch potato he may well be overweight. We all know this is unhealthy but many of us live like this. Obesity, diabetes, and lack of exercise are causally related factors. Researchers have looked at the statistics and are able to evaluate each of these factors independently. They have discovered that each increases the risk of cardiovascular disease. The sum of all three acting together is a multiple risk.

Q If he has one heart attack is he likely to have another?

Yes. A person who has an episode of cardiovascular disease (e.g. a heart attack, angina, or a stroke) is more likely to develop a second (or third) episode.

Q Would regular exercise reduce the risk?

Yes. Regular exercise is very closely linked with a lower incidence of cardiovascular disease. If couch potatoes rise from the sofa three times a week and run 5–6km (2–3 miles), they lower the risk, even if they maintain the same obese weight. One study demonstrated that a group of obese individuals, encouraged by traditional means to regularly exercise and alter their diet, lost an average of one per cent of their body weight.

Q Does drinking coffee increase my risk of heart problems?

Coffee contains caffeine, which increases your heart rate. It may feel as though your heart has a palpitation and skips a beat. Caffeine in other drinks, such as tea, cola, and chocolate, in large enough quantity, can have a similar effect. If your heart is healthy don't worry, but if you've had a heart attack or have other cardiovascular disease, try to cut down on your caffeine intake.

RISK FACTORS FOR CORONARY ARTERY DISEASE

There are a number of risk factors that predispose people to coronary artery disease (CAD) and they can be divided into those you can avoid – or at least modify – and those that are unavoidable because they are inevitable.

AVOIDABLE

Smoking

Stress

Lack of exercise

High blood pressure

High cholesterol

Diabetes (unless inherited)

Obesity

UNAVOIDABLE

Age (growing older)

Gender (being a man or a menopausal woman)

Inherited factors (some people are genetically predisposed to diabetes, heart attacks, or high cholesterol)

The more risk factors you have the more likely you are to develop coronary artery disease. Some, such as smoking and high cholesterol, are more lethal than others.

Increased risk of CAD →

						Lack of exercise
					Stress	Stress
				Obesity	Obesity	Obesity
			Diabetes	Diabetes	Diabetes	Diabetes
		High blood pressure	High blood pressure	High blood pressure	High blood pressure	High blood pressure
	High cholesterol	High cholesterol	High cholesterol	High cholesterol	High cholesterol	High cholesterol
Smoking	Smoking	Smoking	Smoking	Smoking	Smoking	Smoking

Risk factors →

Q Are the heart and emotions linked?

The heart and emotions have always been linked in common parlance. We speak of heartfelt sorrow, the suitor's heart skips a beat when he catches sight of his damsel, he is broken-hearted when she mails him a "Dear John" note, the spirited man is full of heart, and the mean man is heartless. However, whether emotions contribute to heart problems is very difficult to prove scientifically, so the jury is still out.

Q Do strong emotions put my heart at risk?

Possibly. There is an increasing amount of evidence to suggest that emotions, such as anxiety, depression, anger, and even loneliness, when they are long-term and chronic, can contribute to heart problems, either by making them worse or by initiating them in the first place. It's almost as though persistent worry, low self-esteem, moodiness, and lack of motivation eat away at an individual's inside, upsetting the normal regulation of the body's metabolism and the smooth operation of the nervous system. The condition is obviously made worse if such individuals turn to cigarettes and/or alcohol for relief from their woes.

Q In my youth my doctor said I had a Type A personality, which made me prone to heart disease. Is this still true?

Forty or more years ago, it was commonplace to speak of Type A and Type B personalities. The Type A was aggressive, striving, demanding, and even hostile. The reporting investigators claimed that these people had a significantly higher incidence of cardiovascular disease when compared to the Type B personality, who was a laid-back, relaxed individual. However, subsequent investigators have focused more on anxiety, depression and other psychological factors that also corrolate with an increased risk of heart attack.

Q Will a very stressful lifestyle lead to heart disease?

Yes, probably. We can all select the highly anxious, the acutely stressed, or the very depressed from the crowd. However, the majority of us are a bit stressed and somewhat anxious. Do we, too, have a greater incidence of cardiovascular disease? Stress is internalized differently by each of us. The death of Mr Jones' wife might be traumatic for him and yet the death of Mr Smith's wife might affect him less. It has been shown that depression, anxiety, stress, and social isolation are all linked with a higher incidence of cardiovascular disease and hamper ability to recover from the disease.

Q Why are depressed, anxious, stressed, and isolated people linked to cardiovascular problems?

This link raises much speculation and evidence suggests that all these people share a more dismal lifestyle. They tend to eat poorly, perform less exercise, be fatter, less compliant with their medication, smoke more, and consequently develop more cardiovascular problems, yet deal with them less successfully.

Q Does working in a stressful environment increase my risk of a heart attack?

It may, if you carry on working stressfully for a long period of time. We all thrive on a little stress – it's part of modern life – but chronic stress is bad for you. A study published in 2003 in the UK describes how long-term stress can be worse for you than putting on 18kg (40lbs) or being 30 years older, because workers compensate for the stress by drinking more alcohol, smoking more, and failing to exercise. The study showed that a stressful working environment increases the risk of heart attacks and the risk of fatal strokes. Manual workers are particularly at risk, presumably because they tend to work overtime and do night shifts, which disrupt their cycle of sleeping and waking.

Q How does my body respond to stress?

Your body responds in two ways. There's an immediate, short-term response, then a long-term response to persistent stress. The short-term response, known as "fight-or-flight", kicks in as soon you feel threatened or angry: your adrenal glands release adrenaline into the bloodstream, making your breathing and heart rate increase and making more glucose available for your instant energy needs. More blood goes to your brain and muscles so you can think better and move quickly, while less blood goes to your skin and digestive system.

Q And the long-term response to stress?

Prolonged stress causes the adrenal glands, via command signals from the hypothalamus and pituitary gland in your brain, to release cortisol and other hormones into the blood. Over time, these have negative effects that damage your body: for example, blood pressure may increase and kidney function can be affected and may deteriorate over time, increasing the risk of cardiovascular disease. Some research suggests that changes in the blood-clotting mechanism also raises the prospect of a heart attack.

Q Is smoking really such a high risk factor?

Smoking is one of the biggest contributors to developing heart disease. The US Surgeon General has called it "the leading preventable cause of disease and deaths in the United States". Smoking causes coronary artery disease – smokers are 2 to 4 times more likely to develop coronary disease than nonsmokers. As few as 1–4 cigarettes daily triples the risk of heart-related death. Cigarette smoking doubles a person's risk for stroke, reduces circulation, and causes peripheral vascular disease and abdominal aortic aneurysms.

Q Why is smoking so dangerous for my heart and circulation?

Smoke from cigarette, cigars, and pipes contains toxic chemicals, such as tar, carbon monoxide, and nicotine. The tar coats the lining of your lungs and the carbon monoxide makes it harder for your red blood cells to carry oxygen. It binds to the haemoglobin hundreds of times more easily than oxygen does; carbon monoxide from smoking reduces more than an estimated 8 per cent of the oxygen-carrying capacity of the blood. As a result the cardiovascular system has to work harder to deliver the oxygen the cells need, and heart muscle cells do not receive adequate oxygen. One of the effects of nicotine is to stimulate the release of adrenaline, which causes blood pressure to rise. Smoking also causes fatty deposits in the lining of the arteries, which narrows them, increasing the risk of angina and heart attack.

Q What about low-tar cigarettes?

Smoking these cigarettes will not reduce your risk of developing cardiovascular diseases because, while they may create less tar, their smoke still contains other toxic chemicals. Many people who smoke low-tar cigarettes – whether they are "light" or "mild" – are being fooled into thinking that they are not as bad for them as "stronger" cigarettes.

Q Is passive smoking a risk, too?

Yes. However, your risk is not nearly as high as a smoker's. The environmental tobacco smoke, both from burning cigarettes and from the smoke exhaled by smokers, still contains toxic substances that you inhale. Studies have shown that people who live with partners who smoke are at a greater risk of heart disease than people who live in a nonsmoking household.

Myth "Drinking red wine is good for the heart"

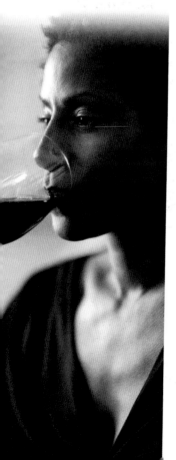

Truth There is a fair amount of evidence to suggest this is true, especially if the red wine is drunk with meals. It is thought that flavonoids, which are found in high levels in red wine, combat the damaging effect of free radicals, which are dangerous molecules that can cause serious problems in the body's cells, including the muscle cells of the heart.

Q **How quickly does my body recover if I give up smoking?**

Stopping smoking is a very effective way to lower the risk of cardiovascular diseases that may otherwise be fatal. As soon as you stop your body starts to repair the damage and in a short time – perhaps within 24 hours – your heart receives substantially more oxygen. And the longer you don't smoke, the more you reduce the risk of cardiovascular diseases.

Q **How much less is the risk of coronary artery disease if I give up smoking?**

Cigarette smoking cessation alone leads to a 36 per cent reduction in the death rate from coronary artery disease, the most prevalent type of cardiovascular disease. In fact, the incidence of non-fatal coronary artery disease is reduced by the same 36 per cent when comparing populations who stopped smoking with those who never smoked.

Q **Would I also be less likely to suffer a stroke?**

The incidence of, and deaths resulting from, strokes is much higher in smokers than in those who have stopped smoking. This is true for the entire spectrum of cardiovascular disease.

Q **What are the negative health effects of drinking alcohol?**

High blood pressure can be caused by regular consumption of more than the daily recommended amount of alcohol (see p145), thereby raising the risk of developing cardiovascular diseases. The heart may perform less efficiently, because alcohol can damage the heart muscle directly, causing the chambers to enlarge and weaken (cardiomyopathy). Drinkers with an enlarged heart may develop signs and symptoms of congestive heart failure such as swollen ankles and shortness of breath. It may also disrupt the heart rhythm most commonly causing atrial fibrillation.

Q Are there any benefits of drinking alcohol?

Yes, several. Well-documented research shows that moderate alcohol consumption (1–2 drinks per day – see p145) is associated with a 30–50 per cent reduction in the risk of developing cardiovascular disease. It may actually protect from coronary artery disease, especially in post-menopausal women and men over the age of 40. More alcohol than recommended, however, increases the risk of heart disease.

Q How do moderate amounts of alcohol protect the heart?

Research suggests that up to 50 per cent of alcohol's protective effect is due to its ability to raise the level of high-density lipoprotein (HDL), the good cholesterol (see p38). Moderate amounts of alcohol may also make the blood less sticky so it flows more smoothly, reducing the chances of developing a heart attack or stroke. These benefits may be maximized when the alcohol is drunk with a meal.

Q What do recreational drugs, such as cocaine, do to the heart?

Cocaine is a stimulant and one of the most widely used recreational drugs. However, it is also one of the most dangerous drugs for the heart. Many other recreational drugs affect the heart. Cocaine can reduce the blood supply to the heart, cause arrythmias, and directly impair heart function.

Q How does cocaine cause this imbalance in blood supply?

Cocaine causes the coronary arteries to constrict while at the same time it stimulates the heart muscle to demand more oxygen, a paradoxical effect. Normally when the heart has an increased demand for oxygen the coronary arteries dilate. Instead, they constrict under the influence of cocaine. The result increases the chances of a heart attack, which could be fatal.

Q What is the likelihood of a cocaine user having a heart attack?

The risk of a heart attack is increased 24 times in the 60 minutes following cocaine use. A heart attack can occur with a first-time user or a habitual abuser. In addition to causing an imbalance in the coronary artery blood supply (see p48), cocaine activates the blood clotting mechanism. Since a clot is often the ultimate step prior to a heart attack, this further increases the risk of a heart attack. They occur most commonly after sniffing cocaine through the nose (the most common route of using cocaine). The mean age of those who sustain a heart attack after cocaine use is 34. Twenty per cent are under the age of 25.

Q Can cocaine use be fatal?

Yes. Although the mechanism is poorly understood, cocaine can lead to cardiac arrhythmias of all types and occasionally they are fatal. Fatal cardiovascular complications after cocaine use are rather uncommon. Death results from cocaine use in less than two per cent of instances. This is probably because cocaine use typically occurs in the young – who do not normally have pre-existing heart diseases.

Q Does the recreational drug ecstasy have any effect on the heart?

Yes. Ecstasy is a drug that contains a psychoactive stimulant known as MDMA. This ingredient primarily has an effect on the brain, but it has been shown to cause high blood pressure and tachycardia (rapid beating of the heart). Very rarely it may severely disrupt the temperature regulation system of the body, an action that jeopardizes the function of the kidneys, liver, and the whole cardiovascular system. Research suggests, however, that ecstasy does not seem to be implicated in coronary artery disease.

Obesity and diabetes

Q How many people are obese?

Obesity is an increasing problem worldwide. Fifty years ago, there was limited knowledge about obesity and it was not felt to be of concern. Now even childhood obesity is making headlines in countries around the world. Figures from The World Health Organization reveal that in 2005 there were approximately 1.6 billion adults who were overweight and around 400 million of them were obese. Predictions for the future indicate that by 2015 there will be more than 2.3 billion overweight adults and 700 million will be obese. The figures are determined using body mass index (BMI), which is a global standardized measure (see pp136–137) that combines weight and height.

Q Why are obese people likely to develop heart disease?

People with obesity are likely to have higher total cholesterol, LDL cholesterol, blood pressure, and C reactive protein (see p91), and thus a higher rate of cardiovascular disease. Obesity is a killer. It cannot be demonstrated that obesity, if isolated from these other factors, is a reliable predictor of cardiovascular disease but that is not inconsequential since it is associated very clearly with all of the factors mentioned that are known precursors of cardiovascular disease.

Q Does weight loss reduce the risk of heart disease?

Yes. Observational studies have shown that weight loss is clearly associated with a lowering of total cholesterol, LDL cholesterol, blood pressure, and C reactive protein. Thus, the incidence of cardiovascular disease is reduced with weight loss. (See weight-loss diet, p147.)

Q Does obesity in childhood increase the risk of heart disease?

Yes. Childhood obesity is a very reliable predictor of later cardiovascular disease. This is particularly concerning since there is a marked increase in the rate of obesity in children and adolescents. According to the International Obesity Task Force, one in ten children between the ages of five and 17 – more than 155 million – around the world are either overweight or obese.

Q What is the risk of heart disease if I have diabetes?

As a general rule, you are two to five times more likely to develop heart disease than normal. Type 2 diabetics tend to have increased levels of fat, such as cholesterol and triglycerides, in their blood. Often, the proportion of HDL and LDL (see pp38–39) is reversed so that more of the bad cholesterol accumulates. As a result, Type 2 diabetes is associated with narrowing of the arteries (atherosclerosis) because blood vessels become scarred and hard plaques (atheromata) form on their inner lining. Thus, diabetics have an increased incidence of strokes, heart attacks, and peripheral vascular disease (atherosclerosis in the legs), as well as many noncardiovascular complications that result from the diffuse vascular effects.

Q What does this mean for diabetics?

The heart muscle of diabetics is more likely to become damaged (cardiomyopathy), and they are more likely to experience a cardiovascular event, such as a heart attack. Their chances of dying from such an event are higher than for non-diabetics. In addition, if they do recover, they are more likely to experience another cardiovascular event at some time in the future.

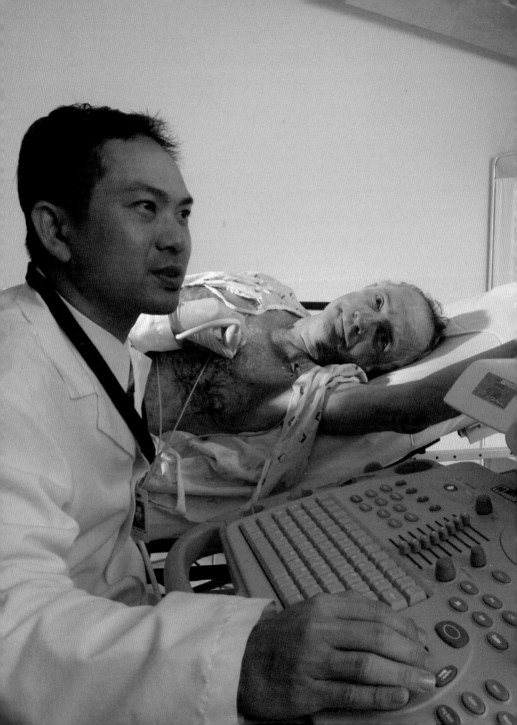

Heart problems

The most common heart problems
are related to four main areas of the
heart's function: insufficient blood
flow through the coronary arteries;
abnormalities of the heart rhythm;
a fault in one or more of the valves;
or abnormal function of the cardiac
muscle. Heart problems may be
inherited or acquired, for instance
resulting from inflammation or
infection, or from environmental
factors such as cigarette smoking.

Coronary artery disease

Q What is coronary artery disease?

This serious disease occurs when the coronary arteries are narrowed or blocked. It is a rather simple concept: a kind of supply-and-demand disorder. The function of these arteries is compromised and their supply of blood to the heart muscle is limited and cannot meet the excess demand when needed. At rest, particularly during sleep, the heart demands little in terms of supply. However, there are times – usually during exercise or stress – when the heart needs to supply more blood to both its own heart muscle and the rest of the body.

Q How common is coronary artery disease?

Coronary artery disease, which is also known as coronary heart disease, has caused more deaths in the last 50 years than any other disorder. Worldwide, millions of people have succumbed to this disease.

Q When does coronary artery disease begin?

Narrowing of the coronary arteries occurs gradually after the process of atherosclerosis (see p56) begins, when fatty deposits accumulate on the inner lining of the arteries. Atherosclerosis typically starts in childhood and progresses with age. Many decades may pass before the process reaches a critical point when the narrowing causes problems with the heart. This point may be reached at any time in life, but usually occurs in later years, when any one of the coronary blood vessels – from the main arteries to the smaller arterioles – becomes obstructed by at least 75 per cent. This causes a significant decrease in blood flow, and can result in symptoms of angina pectoris.

Q **What happens when you get angina pectoris?**

The term angina pectoris derives from the Greek and means "pain in the chest". Typically, you feel this pain in the middle of your chest, beneath your breastbone (sternum). The symptoms can vary, but a frequent characteristic is a feeling of pressure, squeezing, or heaviness, which may radiate into your left arm. Less commonly, it radiates into your jaw or even into your right arm. At times, angina may cause nausea (you may even vomit), shortness of breath, and sweating.

Q **When am I likely to experience an episode of angina?**

Angina is usually associated with some form of exertion – for example, walking, eating a meal, or climbing a flight of stairs – and is relieved as the exertion ceases. In a classic case, the chest discomfort lasts for several minutes and can recur with a repeated exertion.

Q **What should I do to relieve the angina?**

The best thing to do is listen to your body, stop whatever you are doing, and rest. If you are walking, then sit down. If anger has brought on the angina, withdraw from the situation. Make no mistake, your heart has reached its maximum workload and cannot do more, so to continue your exertion may lead to a heart attack.

Q **Could I experience a heart attack rather than angina?**

Yes, if the coronary vessel is totally obstructed instead of partially blocked, you will probably have a heart attack. This is known as a myocardial infarction (MI) as a part of your heart muscle dies (infarcts). It occurs when a blood clot forms on a cholesterol plaque and suddenly blocks the coronary artery supplying an area of heart muscle. How much heart muscle dies depends on where the blockage occurs (see p57) and how rapidly medical care is delivered.

Narrowed arteries

Keeping your blood flowing smoothly and at the right pressure is vital for maintaining a healthy heart and a healthy body. When blood flow in the circulation is interrupted by one or more narrowed arteries, problems in the cardiovascular system start to develop. More importantly, if an artery such as one of the coronary arteries becomes completely blocked, the consequences can be fatal if the blockage is left untreated. The most common reason for narrowed arteries is atherosclerosis (see below).

ATHEROSCLEROSIS

Atherosclerosis is a disease that occurs when fatty substances, such as cholesterol, accumulate on the inner lining of an artery and restrict the smooth flow of blood. In the early stages (right), globules of fat start to settle as yellow fatty deposits called atheroma on the artery's lining. At first, the narrowing is marginal and the flow of blood is only slightly restricted.

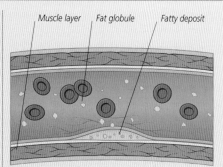

Muscle layer   Fat globule   Fatty deposit

EARLY ATHEROSCLEROSIS

Eventually, the fatty deposits grow larger and the layer of smooth muscle below starts to thicken (right). The artery becomes narrower and the flow of blood restricted. If the atherosclerotic plaque ruptures (cracks) suddenly, blood cells called platelets accumulate on the surface of the atheroma and cause clotting, which may block the artery completely and cause a heart attack.

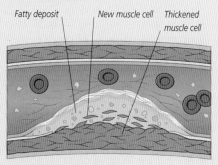

Fatty deposit   New muscle cell   Thickened muscle cell

ADVANCED ATHEROSCLEROSIS

THE STAGES OF CORONARY ARTERY DISEASE

Coronary artery disease develops in stages as atherosclerosis affects the width of the coronary arteries that supply the heart muscles with blood. Normally, the arteries are clear, allowing blood to flow smoothly and the heart muscle cells to receive an adequate supply of nutrients. As fatty deposits form on the lining of an artery, the blood flow is partially blocked. The artery may also become fully blocked (see p54 & 56), cutting off the blood to the muscle cells and damaging them.

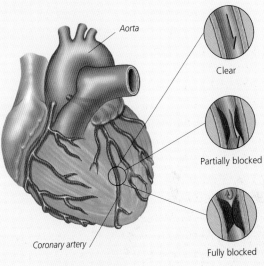

Aorta

Clear

Partially blocked

Coronary artery

Fully blocked

CORONARY ARTERIES

DAMAGE TO HEART MUSCLE

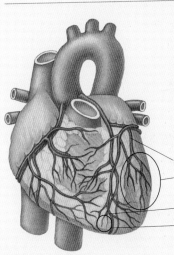

The consequence of a blocked coronary artery can be a very serious heart attack. If the blockage is in a main artery, then the area of heart muscle that is damaged may be very large and the heart attack may be major. However, if the blockage is in a small artery at the end of a branch, then the area of damaged muscle is small and the resulting heart attack more minor.

Site of blockage in a main artery

Area of muscle affected

Site of blockage in a small artery

Area of muscle affected

AREAS OF AFFECTED HEART MUSCLE

HEART ATTACKS

Some people who are at risk of coronary artery disease may have been warned by their doctor that they may experience a heart attack. They may have some idea what to expect and what to do if it happens. Others, especially those who have had no history of heart problems, have no warning whatsoever and may even confuse the symptoms of a heart attack with other causes.

WHAT A HEART ATTACK FEELS LIKE

When you have a myocardial infarction, the symptoms of chest discomfort can be quite similar to those of angina pectoris described on p55. However, the discomfort is typically more severe, lasts longer than the few minutes of angina, and has more intense constitutional symptoms, such as breathlessness, nausea, vomiting, and sweating. A myocardial infarction is not necessarily related to exertion and can present with unusual symptoms or none at all.

TAKING ACTION

If you have a heart attack you must get medical help at once (see p94). If someone is experiencing what looks like a heart attack, he or she needs to go to a hospital – or at least receive immediate attention from a paramedic. At the hospital the patient will be taken to the emergency room or a cardiac care unit, at least for observation. If the diagnosis is coronary artery disease in which the coronary circulation has been compromised, the necessary steps can be taken to ameliorate the situation and preserve as much viable heart muscle as possible. The longer you wait to seek medical attention, the less heart muscle will be able to be salvaged.

OTHER CAUSES OF CHEST PAIN

There are several alternative causes of chest pain that are not related to poor blood supply to the heart. If you feel a sharp pain when you inhale (pleuritic chest pain) you may have a pneumonia or a pulmonary embolism (blood clot to the lung). Alternatively, it could be a musculoskeletal pain caused by an injury or a pain in the left chest area from a shingles infection. A burning pain under the breastbone may be associated with gastro-oesophageal reflux disease, in which stomach acid flows back into the oesophagus.

Q Can a blood clot cause a heart attack?

Yes. Aside from the gradual process of atherosclerosis that leads to progressive narrowing of a coronary artery or smaller vessel, blood clots play an important role in the genesis of a heart attack because they can form a blockage and prevent the supply of blood to the heart muscle. There are two kinds of clot – an embolus, which breaks off from a clot formed elsewhere in the body and travels around in the blood, and a thrombus, which remains in and blocks the vessel where it was formed.

Q Where does an embolus come from?

An embolus can reach the blood vessels in the coronary circulation from a pre-existing clot in either the left atrium or the left ventricle. It can also come from a blood clot formed on a heart valve that has been infected in endocarditis (see p76–77), in which the lining of the heart is inflamed after invasion by bacteria.

Q How does a thrombus form?

Thromboses (the plural of thrombus) are the more common form of blood clot involved in ischemic heart disease. When a coronary artery or smaller vessel has been affected by atherosclerosis (see p56), a thrombus may form at the site of maximal narrowing and this can cause a heart attack. If an atherosclerotic plaque ruptures, then a thrombus may form, causing the complete obstruction of a coronary blood vessel that was only minimally narrowed before. This is the most common cause of heart attack.

Q What is the result of a complete blockage?

When any branch of a coronary artery is totally blocked (occluded) a myocardial infarction follows, because the part of heart muscle supplied by that part of the artery is denied its blood supply and thus dies (see p57).

Arrhythmias

Q What are arrhythmias?

These are disorders of the heart's normal rhythm (see pp20–21), called normal sinus rhythm, when the heart beats between 60 and 100 times per minute. The heart beat is regular in a sinus rhythm. In other words, the time that elapses between each heartbeat is virtually the same. Each regular sinus beat originates in the sinoatrial (SA) node in the right atrium of the heart. When the rhythm deviates from the normal, the result is an arrhythmia. There are three main types of arrhythmia – atrial arrhythmias, ventricular arrhythmias, and atrioventricular block.

Q Can my heart rhythm be normal if my heart rate is too slow or too fast?

Yes, as long as all the criteria satisfy the definition of sinus rhythm (see above). If your heart rate is below 60 beats per minute while in sinus rhythm, it is referred to as sinus bradycardia ("brady" means "slow"). If, on the other hand, sinus conditions prevail but your heart rate has risen above 100 beats per minute, this is referred to as sinus tachycardia ("tachy" means "fast"). These are both normal rhythms.

Q I have been diagnosed with a sinus arrhythmia. What is this?

This is a normal heart rhythm. It is the term used to define slight variations in heart rate when the heart is in sinus rhythm. It occurs most commonly in children and young adults, and is frequently exacerbated by the breathing cycle. This form of variation in heart rate is not associated with any particular heart disease, nor does it lead to any heart problems. Technically, it is not even considered an arrhythmia.

Q Is sick sinus syndrome different to sinus arrhythmia?

Yes. Sick sinus syndrome refers to a condition which can produce potentially serious symptoms. Basically, the SA node functions unreliably. Characteristically, the heart rate varies between going too slowly and too rapidly. There may be sinus pauses where the SA node fails to discharge (or fails to trigger the atria) for a few seconds. These can be followed by rapid rates that may reach 200 beats per minute for several seconds.

Q My mother has been diagnosed with an atrial arrhythmia. What is this?

An atrial arrhythmia is any abnormal heart rhythm that starts in the atrium. The most common atrial arrhythmia is when the heartbeat is triggered by atrial premature contractions (APCs). This can occur in people with no underlying heart disease, but may also be seen in the presence of a cardiac condition. Normally, the cells in the SA node initiate contractions in the atria and then, for a short time after, do not respond even if there is another electrical impulse. To trigger an APC, a heart cell in the atrium outside the SA node initiates an early contraction. APCs can be exacerbated by caffeine intake.

Q Do I have a heart problem if my heart flutters?

Possibly. An occasional palpitation or flutter can simply indicate a benign atrial premature contraction (APC). Longer bouts of heart fluttering may reflect atrial flutter, an atrial arrhythmia in which the atria beat in a rapid, regular fashion 250 to 350 times per minute. Typically, there is a normal blocking action at the AV node so that only one in two of the atrial beats is transmitted to the ventricles. Thus, with this so-called 2:1 block, the ventricular (pulse) rate is 150 beats per minute. Atrial flutter is seen in several cardiac diseases, but can occur in an otherwise normal heart.

Myth "Heart disease is a part of growing old"

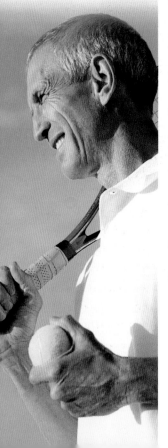

Truth But if you look after yourself, eat a heart-healthy diet, and exercise regularly, then this is not entirely correct. Of course, the normal wear and tear of ageing body tissues exposes your heart and circulation to problems, and this can be made worse – and perhaps even inevitable – by bad habits, such as smoking and drinking alcohol, and worrying too much about stressful situations.

Q What is happening when a heart seems to quiver instead of beating regularly?

This is called atrial fibrillation (A fib). It is remarkably common, occurring in 1 per cent of people over 60, and increasing to 5 per cent of people over 69. In A fib the atria trigger disorganizes electrical impulses between 400 and 600 times a minute, too rapidly for the atria to effectively contract, so they virtually quiver in an irregular fashion. The AV node is bombarded by this rapid onslaught of impulses, but does not allow all of them to pass through to the ventricles. Typically, 110–150 impulses each minute do excite the ventricles to beat in a rhythm described as irregularly irregular. This rhythm lacks any order whatsoever. A fib may cause symptoms such as light-headedness or palpitations, or may occur without symptoms.

Q What happens when a heart speeds up in short bursts, then suddenly returns to normal?

This is probably a supraventricular tachycardia (SVT), which is an arrhythmia that arises in the atria. The rate is typically 150 to 200 beats per minute. Very often, the arrythmia occurs in recurrent short bursts that stop spontaneously. Treatment is only considered necessary if episodes are frequent or cause discomfort.

Q Caffeine seems to make my heart beat oddly. What could this be?

Caffeine commonly causes atrial premature contractions (APCs, see p61). Alternatively, you could be feeling ventricular premature contractions (VPCs), which is when your ventricles contract a little early in the cardiac cycle. VPCs are quite common, particularly in children and teenagers. There is usually no underlying heart problem, but occasionally VPCs can be caused by underlying heart damage, so your doctor may recommend tests to determine if your heart is healthy. Other substances that cause VPCs include tobacco and alcohol.

Q My doctor said I had an episode of ventricular tachycardia. Is that a serious problem?

Yes. Ventricular tachycardia (VT) is a potentially fatal arrhythmia that occurs when VPCs are sustained for 30 or more seconds. The heart rate varies but is predominantly very fast (up to 250 beats per minute). The heartbeat is so rapid that the ventricles do not have time to fill with blood before they contract, so the heart is unable to pump adequate blood flow to the body. This results in light-headedness, and can lead to loss of consciousness and cardiac arrest. VT is treated with an implanted cardioverter defibrillator and drugs to prevent a recurrence.

Q Is ventricular tachycardia (VT) associated with heart disease?

Yes. Over half of the patients who develop VT have underlying coronary artery disease and most others have alternate forms of heart disease. Very few have no underlying heart disease. Symptoms depend on the rate and duration of the VT. If the rate is excessive, as is typically the case, the cardiac output is inadequate and cardiovascular collapse might follow. However, if the VT is brief and spontaneously remits, symptoms are either absent or, at most, brief and mild.

Q What causes sudden death?

Sudden death is most frequently attributed to ventricular fibrillation (VF). This arrhythmia causes the ventricles to quiver at rates in excess of 300 oscillations per minute. Such ventricular activity cannot sustain organized contractions needed to circulate blood, so death follows in minutes unless corrective action – direct-current (DC) cardioversion (see p95) – is taken. Those people who survive VF need an implantable cardioverter defibrillator (see p95) to instantaneously treat a potential recurrence.

HEART RHYTHMS

The normal rhythmic beating of the heart is triggered by a pacemaker called the sinoatrial (SA) node in the right atrium (see p20). If the rhythm of the electrical output of the sinoatrial node becomes irregular, then the heartbeat becomes abnormal.

Abnormal heart rhythms may be short-lived and cause no harm. Sometimes they are more serious and need medical attention. An electrocardiogram or ECG (see pp82–85) shows what happens to the heartbeat in two examples – sinus tachycardia and atrial fibrillation – when compared to a normal heart.

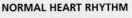

NORMAL HEART RHYTHM
The normal ECG pattern shows a small peak as the atria contract, a large peak as the ventricles contract, and a third peak as the ventricles relax.

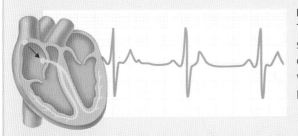

SINUS TACHYCARDIA
A speeded-up rhythm from the sinoatrial node makes the heart beat 30 times more per minute than normal. The ECG shows the peaks are much closer together.

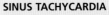

ATRIAL FIBRILLATION
A chaotic rhythm is triggered from many areas in the atrium of which only few impulses reach the ventricles. A fib makes the atria contract inefficiently and very rapidly.

Q What happens if the electrical impulse fails to reach the ventricular tissue?

This is called atrioventricular (AV) block. There are three kinds: first-, second-, and third-degree AV block. In a first-degree block, all beats are conducted from the atria to the ventricles, but with a delay in the normal conduction time. In a second-degree block, not all the beats are successfully conducted from the atria to the ventricles, causing "dropped beats". Third-degree block, or complete heart block, means no impulses are conducted from the atria to the ventricles so that they operate independently of one another. The SA node continues to trigger atrial contraction, and secondary pacemakers in the ventricle trigger slow ventricular contractions.

Q If I have AV block, is it associated with underlying heart disease?

Yes. Most instances of second- and third-degree AV block are linked to an underlying disease, typically ischemic heart disease. They are common in the elderly, as ageing affects the conducting system, or can be caused by medications or injury after heart surgery. Complete heart block can be an emergency requiring a pacemaker (see p112).

Q In general, should arrhythmias be treated or left alone?

Arrhythmias are common, yet few need any treatment and are left alone. Sometimes treatment is mandatory. For example, a pacemaker (see p112) is required in complete heart block and anticoagulation in atrial fibrillation (see p113). Ventricular fibrillation (see p64) and ventricular tachycardia are treated with electrical cardioversion (see p95), and an implantable cardioverter defibrillator. However, the more common arrhythmias – for example, atrial and ventricular premature contractions – do not usually need treatment and often settle spontaneously.

Valve disorders

Q My daughter has been diagnosed with mitral stenosis –what is this?

The opening of the mitral valve (see p16) in her heart is narrowed and restricts the flow of blood from the left atrium into the left ventricle. Normally, the cross-sectional area of the valve is reduced to below 1.5sq cm (0.23sq in) before symptoms develop.

Q What is the effect of this stenosis?

Blood pressure in the atrium increases, affecting the pressure in the lungs, which causes shortness of breath. The left atrium increases in size to compensate. This may lead to atrial arrhythmias, typically atrial fibrillation (see p63).

Q What could have caused my daughter's ailment?

It is most commonly caused by a rare childhood infection called acute rheumatic fever. When the heart is involved, it is called rheumatic heart disease. The cusps of the affected valve, and the chordae tendinae and papillary muscles that anchor the cusps, can become inflamed, scarred, and shortened.

Q Can the mitral valve develop a leak?

Yes. When the valve doesn't close fully it is referred to as incompetent, and the leak is known as mitral regurgitation. Since blood flows backward into the upper chamber, over time the heart has to work harder, which can result in heart failure. You then become breathless and develop fluid retention. One common cause is a called mitral valve prolapse. Other causes are infective endocarditis (see pp76–77) or a damaged heart muscle. An echocardiogram (see p84) can diagnose mitral regurgitation and surgery can fix it.

Q What is aortic stenosis?

Aortic stenosis is the narrowing of the aortic valve, which reduces the blood flow from the heart to the rest of the body. The left ventricle enlarges as a result of the strain of pumping against the blocked valve. After some time, you may develop angina or feel faint (due to an inadequate supply of blood to the brain). Congestive heart failure (see p73) may ultimately result from left ventricular strain, so it is essential to fix the aortic valve to prevent progression of the disease. Aortic stenosis requires surgery, and can be fatal if left untreated.

Q How can I develop aortic stenosis?

The most common cause today is from a degenerative heart disease that occurs more commonly in old people. It involves the valve commissures (the connecting areas between the cusps), which stick together, fuse, and finally accumulate calcium deposits. This condition can be congenital or caused by rheumatic heart disease.

Q Can my aortic valve leak?

Yes. When this happens, some of the blood pumped into the aorta leaks (regurgitates) back into the left ventricle, which is forced to work overtime to accommodate the extra blood. The ventricle thickens in response to the extra strain, then enlarges (dilates). The strain generates increased pressure in the left ventricle and is transmitted back to the left atrium and to the lungs, which can fill with fluid so that you may become short of breath. The failure of the left ventricle can eventually cause the right ventricle to fail as well, if the disease progresses without appropriate treatment.

ABNORMAL VALVES

The four valves in the heart (see pp15–17) ensure that blood flows in one direction only. They open fully to allow blood to pass through, then close completely when the muscles of the heart contract. If either of these functions fails, the efficiency of the heart is impaired.

VALVE STENOSIS

The cusps of a normal, healthy valve are flexible and freely open to their full extent to let the blood pass through. Cusps that are stiff or narrow do not open fully, restricting the blood flow and putting a strain on the heart. Such cusps are called "stenosed."

VALVE INCOMPETENCE

When they close, the cusps of a normal, healthy valve fit tightly together and prevent blood from flowing back. Cusps that do not close tightly are known as "incompetent". They allow blood to leak back (or regurgitate), which forces the heart to work harder.

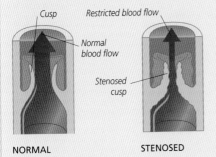

Cusp   Restricted blood flow
Normal blood flow
Stenosed cusp

NORMAL   STENOSED

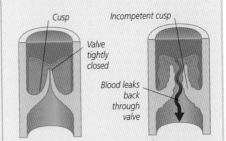

Cusp   Incompetent cusp
Valve tightly closed
Blood leaks back through valve

NORMAL   INCOMPETENT

THE PULMONARY VALVE

The three cusps of the pulmonary valve are rounded underneath and fit tightly together when they are closed. As a result, they completely seal the entrance between the right ventricle and the pulmonary artery. The pulmonary valve rarely develops stenosis or becomes incompetent.

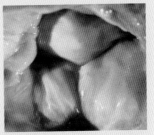

CLOSED PULMONARY VALVE

Q Can a leaky aortic valve be fixed?

Yes. Symptoms develop once the leaking becomes severe and the ventricle becomes weakened, causing heart failure. It is important to detect a leaky valve early by physical examination and ultrasound, since medication can slow progression of the disease. Once the leaking is significant, aortic valve replacement is the treatment of choice (see p120).

Q Can my tricuspid valve develop stenosis?

Yes, but usually from rheumatic fever, which is rare, except in developing countries. Typically, the mitral valve is also affected.

Q What happens as a result of tricuspid stenosis?

Stenosis of the tricuspid valve ultimately leads to heart failure and accumulation of fluid in the body. Since the circulating blood from your body is restricted by the valve, the cardiac output diminishes and fatigue becomes a progressive problem. Treatment is surgical with a tricuspid valve replacement.

Q Is my pulmonary valve likely to develop stenosis?

Stenosis of the pulmonary valve may develop but is uncommon. It is usually a congenital abnormality that is best managed by dilating the narrowed pulmonary valve with a balloon procedure similar to that used in angioplasty (see pp98–99).

Q Can my pulmonary valve become leaky?

Yes. Pulmonary regurgitation develops mostly in response to high blood pressure in the pulmonary circulation (pulmonary hypertension). The increased workload for the right ventricle reduces its ability to pump blood effectively, causing right-sided heart failure. Symptoms would include fatigue, fluid accumulation, shortness of breath, chest pain, and fainting with exercise.

Heart failure

What is heart failure? Heart failure is a syndrome caused by insufficient blood flow to the body. This typically occurs when the heart muscle is either weak, damaged, or abnormally thick, and therefore too inefficient to pump an adequate supply of blood to the organs and muscles. In the absence of sufficient blood flow, which deprives the body of crucial oxygen, glucose, and nutrients, over time the muscles can become weak and the organs may become unable to function properly.

What are the effects of heart failure? The body attempts to compensate for the weakened heart muscle by increasing the heart rate and raising blood pressure by constricting the blood vessels. This further worsens the function of the heart muscle and contributes to the progression of heart failure syndrome itself. Even the fluid accumulation that is commonly seen in heart failure is the result of the body trying to compensate for the reduced blood flow.

How likely am I to develop heart failure? Heart failure is increasingly common. The number of people with heart failure continues to grow, in large part because the treatments for heart problems that frequently used to be fatal, such as heart attacks, have improved to the extent that people survive but may be left with varying degrees of damage to the heart muscle. The likelihood of developing heart failure increases with age, approximately doubling with each decade of life. So as people live longer, the incidence of heart failure continues to increase.

Q Is having heart failure serious?

Yes, but many people with heart failure have no symptoms and lead productive lives once they are on effective treatment. However, life expectancy is reduced so you need to remain under close medical supervision. Fortunately, many therapies and interventions can prolong survival and reduce symptoms.

Q Do all people with heart failure have weakened heart muscle?

No. Heart failure does not always indicate that there is weakened heart muscle, despite the popular image of the "failing heart". In fact, heart failure can also be caused by a thickening of the heart muscle, called hypertrophy, and can occur despite robust heart pumping. Once the normal geometry of the heart is altered, however, even if only thickened, the heart muscle will weaken and dilate over time if untreated. Eventually, even heart failure with normal heart muscle pumping will progress to a weakened and dilated heart.

ACUTE HEART FAILURE

Acute heart failure occurs when the heart suddenly stops pumping efficiently after a sudden large injury such as a major heart attack. As a result, oxygen-rich blood backs up in the pulmonary veins and the pressure makes fluid collect rapidly in both lungs, causing sudden shortness of breath. Fluid in the lungs is called pulmonary oedema (right) and must be treated at once.

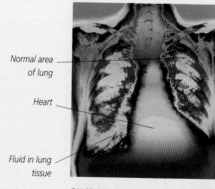

Normal area of lung

Heart

Fluid in lung tissue

FALSE-COLOUR X-RAY SHOWS OEDEMA

Q What causes heart failure?

Coronary artery disease, typically after one or more heart attacks, is the most common cause; high blood pressure the second. Any form of valvular heart disease can also result in heart failure if not treated in time to prevent muscle damage. Some viruses and diseases that cause inflammation can result in heart failure, as can the damage caused by alcohol, illicit drugs, and lead. Peripartum cardiomyopathy, which occurs in the late stages of pregnancy or soon after delivery, can also cause heart failure. Even a chronic, persistently rapid heart rate (tachycardia) can cause heart failure. Commonly, however, the underlying cause remains unknown (idiopathic).

Q Can I inherit heart failure?

Yes. Familial, or inherited, causes of heart failure are increasingly recognized, and probably play a more common role in causing heart failure than previously suspected. Doctors estimate that genetic factors may contribute to up to 50 per cent of such cases.

Q What are the common symptoms of heart failure?

There are many signs and symptoms, any of which can indicate heart failure. Fluid congestion leads to swelling (oedema) in the legs, feet, or abdomen. Shortness of breath can occur with exertion, and even at rest. Waking from sleep with shortness of breath is also a classic sign of progressive heart failure. A night-time cough due to fluid congestion, even in the absence of fluid in the lungs, should not be confused with a passing cough or cold, but should trigger a call to the doctor. Symptoms such as fatigue, chest pain or pressure, and weight gain are also common, as are light-headedness and dizziness.

Q How can my doctor know if I have heart failure?

Many tests can confirm the presence of heart failure. A chest X-ray is a good screening tool for revealing an enlarged heart, and may be the first indication that the heart needs further evaluation. An echocardiogram (see p84) is commonly used for initial diagnosis and then to follow progression of heart function. Heart scans with radioactive tracers, with or without stress tests, are often performed to determine the extent of damage to heart muscle function, and to indicate whether coronary artery disease may be causing the weakened heart muscle. Cardiopulmonary stress tests measure the extent to which exertion is limited by heart failure. CT scans, MRI scans, cardiac catheterizations, and coronary angiograms can also be useful.

Q I feel fine, so why does my doctor say I have heart failure?

Not everyone who has heart failure displays symptoms. In fact, many have few symptoms or signs of the disease, and lead active lifestyles. Contrary to popular belief, there is no direct correlation between the severity of muscle damage and the presence or severity of heart failure symptoms. It is important, however, that you seek medical attention even in the absence of symptoms in order to delay and minimize progression of the disease.

Q Can my stomach pains be caused by heart failure?

It is possible for heart failure only to show itself through symptoms of stomach pains, indigestion, or bloating. Although these abdominal symptoms are more common as the disease progresses, they may be the first symptoms of the disease in both young adults and children. Often this leads doctors to investigate the gastrointestinal system, where findings are usually negative.

Q Can heart failure improve, or can heart muscle recover?

It is often possible to improve the symptoms of heart failure by optimizing medical therapies, exercise, and diet. Some therapies can also improve the heart muscle function itself, to a degree. Having said that, there are some types of damaged heart muscle that can improve, and sometimes even normalize. For instance, heart damage caused by a toxin, such as alcohol, may improve or resolve completely – depending on how long the heart has been exposed to the toxin – when alcohol intake is stopped. Viral causes of heart failure, although potentially fatal, are also potentially reversible.

Q If I have heart failure, what's the best way forward?

Successful treatment of heart failure (see pp115–117) is a team effort of which you are a vital part. You need to get involved and work on changing your lifestyle. In addition, regular follow-ups with your doctor and cardiologist are essential since the team approach, including active participation on the part of the patient, can be very effective in managing this chronic illness.

Q How can I help myself if I have heart failure?

A healthy lifestyle is essential. This includes careful attention to maintaining a low-salt diet (see p150) to minimize fluid retention in your body. You should keep a daily record of your weight to track early signs of fluid retention even before symptoms progress.

Q Is regular exercise important, too?

Yes. In the past it was thought that a sedentary lifestyle was best for heart failure, but it is now well known that regular, moderate exercise is essential. This can include, for example, walking, or riding an exercise bike for 20–30 minutes once or twice daily to optimize the cardiovascular system.

Endocarditis

Q Can my heart catch an infection?

Yes. The most common form is infective endocarditis and is caused by bacteria invading the internal lining of the heart (endocardium), typically involving the heart valves. There are two forms – subacute and acute.

Q How do the bacteria get into the heart to cause an infection?

At first, both the fibrin and platelets in the blood lodge on the surface of a diseased or artificial valve (or other structure). Bacteria in the blood (bacteremia) join a platelet/fibrin mixture to create a vegetation. Bacteremia is common with dental procedures – and even with teeth brushing or vigorous chewing – when small blood vessels are broken. It also occurs when the gut is examined in upper endoscopy or colonoscopy.

Q What are the symptoms of subacute endocarditis?

The classic illness develops over a period of weeks to months and most often affects the mitral and aortic valves in the left side of the heart. The symptoms are vague and felt throughout the body, and are nearly always accompanied by a low-grade fever. The patient may experience fatigue, and loss of appetite and weight. The spleen enlarges, and anaemia develops, as do heart murmurs and frequently tiny bleeding spots in the skin (petechiae) and the nail beds (splinter haemorrhages).

Q Why does the infection lodge in the heart?

Infection usually affects a damaged valve, such as in congenital valve disorders or degenerative valve disease in older patients. Artificial heart valves are also susceptible.

Q How does acute endocarditis differ from the subacute form?

Acute endocarditis is commonly caused by blood infections due to intravenous drug use. It develops quickly in days and usually affects the tricuspid valve, often complicated by infected emboli in the lungs. Staphylococcus aureus is the organism most commonly involved. It is more destructive to tissue and has a higher mortality rate than other bacteria.

Q Does acute endocarditis affect artificial valves?

Endocarditis of artificial valves may occur in up to 20 per cent of all cases of endocarditis. The risk is highest in the first year, but remains higher than normal thereafter. Rarely, bacteria are introduced during surgery. Other causes of bacteremia (see p76) are likely culprits. Infected venous catheters and haemodialysis catheters may also be the cause.

Q How do doctors diagnose endocarditis?

Three separate cultures are taken from the blood over a 24-hour period. If endocarditis is present, the cultures are positive for bacteria in over 95 per cent of cases. A trans-oesophageal echocardiogram (see p85) will identify the valve abnormality and the vegetation in many cases.

Q Is endocarditis fatal and can it be prevented?

This disorder was always fatal in the pre-antibiotic era. Today, the death rate is about 20 per cent and depends on various factors including age, duration of infection, type of infecting bacteria, and presence of artificial valve. Prevention of endocarditis is simple and effective, particularly in dental procedures where patients who are undergoing treatment may be instructed to take an oral antibiotic prophylaxis one hour prior to the procedure. Check with your doctor to see if you are a candidate for this type of antibiotic prophylactic treatment.

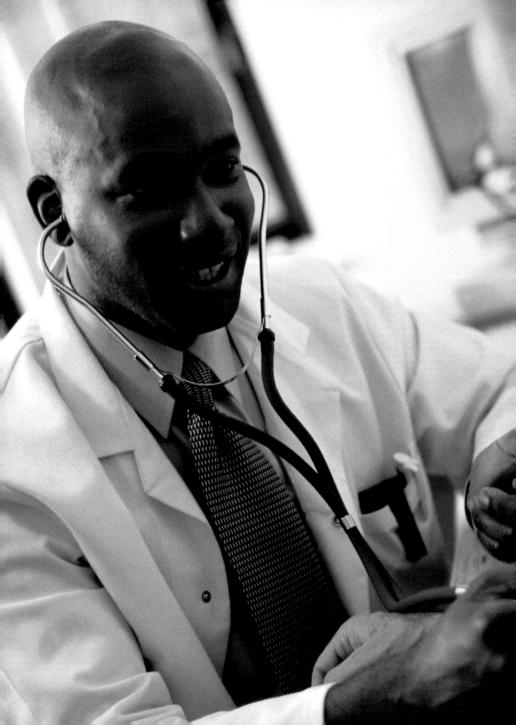

Diagnosing heart problems

Advances in technology and early monitoring of potential problems have led to improved diagnosis of heart disease. If you think you are at risk of a heart problem, discuss your concerns with your doctor, who will take your blood pressure, check your blood for markers, and recommend tests such as electrocardiography, echocardiography, and angiography when appropriate.

Measuring blood pressure

Q How is my blood pressure measured?

A nurse or doctor wraps a cuff around your upper arm and then inflates it manually until no blood flows into your arm. Then air is slowly let out until blood starts to flow, which your nurse hears through a stethoscope placed over an artery in your arm. The cuff is attached to a pressure gauge, which provides the two readings of your blood pressure (see p22).

Q What does the nurse detect with the stethoscope and what does it mean?

The nurse listens for the first sound of the blood flow and notes the corresponding height on the column of mercury. This is the systolic blood pressure (see p22), equivalent to the pressure the heart exerts as the left ventricle contracts. The nurse then listens for the sounds to disappear, again noting the corresponding height of mercury. This reading is the diastolic blood pressure which corresponds to the pressure in the arteries when the heart is at rest.

Q Are there more modern devices?

In many places, modern technology has replaced the manual pumping and the stethoscope with an electronic device that displays your blood pressure digitally.

Q What defines high blood pressure?

Blood pressure is given as one number (the systolic) over another (diastolic) – 120/80mm Hg is typical. Current thinking labels 120–139 (systolic) and 80–89 (diastolic) as prehypertensive and merits further observation. High blood pressure (hypertension) is currently defined as 140/90 or higher for the general population.

Q How does a doctor tell if my blood pressure is elevated?

You need to have several blood pressure readings and calculate the average before a diagnosis of hypertension can be made. In itself, one elevated measure does not define hypertension. Moreover, when your doctor takes your blood pressure it is probably about 10/5mm Hg higher than if it was taken casually at home, perhaps because you're a little stressed about the test.

Q Can I have a blood pressure monitoring machine at home?

Yes, you can buy a semi-automatic device for home use. However, before you buy one ask your doctor which monitoring machines are the most accurate and reliable, and find out how to operate it before taking any readings. A machine at home lets you take multiple measurements that you can show to your doctor, who will confirm or deny a diagnosis of hypertension.

Q Is there a device that takes blood pressure as I walk around?

In special cases, you may be able to wear an ambulatory blood pressure monitor, which measures blood pressure as you walk around. It is not too cumbersome and will record blood pressure readings over a 24-hour period.

Q When should I take my reading?

Blood pressure varies through the day and night, so try several readings over the course of the day. Your blood pressure will be affected by medication, and by stress, so sit down and relax for ten minutes before taking a reading.

Q How often do I need to have my blood pressure taken?

Everyone should have their blood pressure taken once a year as part of a check-up. If you have hypertension you may need to have yours taken every month or so – for example, to keep a watchful eye on the progress of treatment. As soon as your blood pressure stabilizes you may need a measurement every 3–6 months.

Devices to assess the heart

Q How can you tell whether or not my heart is healthy?

Generally, cardiologists use two standard electronic devices to check that your heart is working properly or whether there is some kind of abnormality that needs to be investigated further. First is the electrocardiogram and the other is the echocardiogram (see p84).

Q What is an electrocardiogram?

The electrocardiogram, or ECG, is a very useful tool for measuring the electrical activity of the heart and its muscle cells. It reveals all kinds of information about the health of your heart – contractions, rate, and rhythms – and is important for the diagnosis of a number of heart conditions. It produces a continuous diagram, or trace, of the sequential electrical activity of the heart cells as they cause the heart to beat. The electrocardiogram was invented about 100 years ago by a German scientist and in German it is called an *elektrokardiogramm*, or EKG.

Q I'm due to have an electrocardiogram soon, so what does it involve?

You don't have be be admitted to the hospital for an ECG because the test only takes about ten minutes. You lie down and a technician attaches a number of electrodes in sticky pads to your skin, mostly across your chest, but also two on your arms and legs. Men with hairy chests may have a small area shaved. The ECG trace will be taken when you are resting.

Q Is there an ECG test for angina?

To investigate causes of angina symptoms, you may have an exercise ECG. This test records your heart's activity while you are walking, or cycling on an exercise bike.

Q **What does an ECG measure?**

An ECG is an accurate representation of the time course of the electrical activity of the heart. Thus, it precisely measures the time that elapses as the activity spreads through a chamber and from one chamber to another. It reliably records the rhythm of the heart and assesses the state of the heart's cells.

Q **What does an ECG reveal?**

This is quite complicated. The initial electrical activity starts in the sinoatrial (SA) node (see pp20–21) and spreads to both atria. On an ECG this wave is called the P wave. The impulse travels to the atrioventricular (AV) node, where transmission is delayed momentarily before moving on to both ventricles and causing them to contract. On an ECG you see this as the QRS wave. This is followed by the T wave, which represents a realignment of the electrical charges so that they can discharge again (this is the repolarization wave).

TAKING AN ELECTROCARDIOGRAM

The safe and painless procedure for taking an electrocardiogram (ECG) involves a technician fitting electrodes to the chest to pick up the heart's electrical activity and transmit it to an ECG machine, which prints out a trace.

The printout of an ECG trace shows the electrical activity in one area of the heart. Peaks and troughs reveal the precise moments when the atria and ventricles contract, and when the heart relaxes.

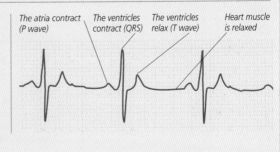

The atria contract (P wave)   *The ventricles contract (QRS)*   *The ventricles relax (T wave)*   *Heart muscle is relaxed*

Q Is an ECG always abnormal during or after a heart attack?

No. Often, the ECG can reveal various characteristic abnormalities that suggest the presence of an acute (or old) heart attack, but the ECG can occasionally be perfectly normal during or after a heart attack.

Q What are some of the other conditions that an ECG can diagnose?

An ECG is a useful tool for detecting arrhythmias (see pp60–66) because it reliably measures the way electrical conduction accelerates or is delayed within chambers or between chambers. When a chamber is enlarged or under strain, or when the heart is affected by certain medications, the ECG may demonstrate characteristic patterns.

Q What is an echocardiogram?

An echocardiogram is an ultrasound device that provides images of the heart's structures on a screen. Ultrasonic waves bounce off an object, such as the left ventricle, and their echo is translated into an image.

TAKING AN ECHOCARDIOGRAM

ECHOCARDIOGRAM OF HEART AND BLOOD FLOW
Echocardiograms are used to look at the chambers and the valves inside the heart using ultrasound waves. The size and function of the heart can be measured from the moving image of a beating heart. The echo indicates the direction of the flow of blood by generating different colours, and detects turbulence that might suggest a valve problem.

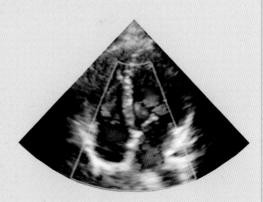

Q If I have an echocardiogram what does it involve?

You will go to a cardiologist's office or hospital, where you lie down in a darkened room so the technician can see the screen. Jelly spread over your chest allows optimal transmission of the ultrasound rays through the skin. The echocardiogram takes about 20–30 minutes and you can watch it on the screen.

Q Do some echocardiograms require patients to swallow a tube?

Yes. This is a trans-oesophageal echocardiogram that takes pictures from the oesophagus directly next to the heart and provides significantly more detail about valves and clots. Even though the tube is small it is unpleasant so you are given a drug to help you relax and a local anaesthetic.

Q What does an echocardiogram assess?

The echocardiogram accurately represents the heart's anatomy and the function of its components, and is particularly useful for diagnosing valve disease.

Q Does an echocardiogram have a value in ischemic heart disease?

Yes. By assessing the way in which the muscular walls of the ventricles contract, the echocardiogram can determine the degree of damage and the overall function of the ventricles. It can also be used in combination with a stress test to diagnose the presence of coronary artery disease.

Q Does an echocardiogram have other diagnostic features?

An echocardiogram is invaluable in diagnosing congenital heart disease, even while the baby is in the womb. The effects of other diseases on the heart, such as high blood pressure, can also be determined. For example, an echocardiogram can estimate the degree of ventricular wall thickening that develops from sustained high blood pressure.

Myth "After the age of 55 women have higher blood pressure than men"

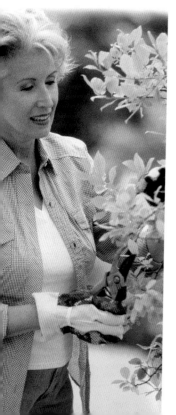

Truth Blood pressure increases with age. Although men have a higher risk of developing high blood pressure than women in their 30s and early 40s, the risk becomes essentially equal for both genders between the ages of 45 and 55. After the age of 55, women are more likely to develop hypertension than men.

Coronary angiograms

Q What is a coronary angiogram?

This is a very useful test that uses a special X-ray technique to directly visualize the anatomy of the coronary arteries (see p88). The most important diagnostic use for coronary angiograms is to detect narrowing of the coronary arteries that results from progressive atherosclerosis (see pp56–57). A coronary angiogram is considered the "gold standard" and all other techniques are measured by it.

Q I am due to have a coronary angiogram soon – what does it involve?

This test involves going to hospital, but does not require an overnight stay. The test usually takes place in the cardiac catheterization laboratory. You will have to avoid food and drink for four hours or so beforehand, as the dye may make you feel nauseous. You may be offered a drug to help you relax, and a local anaesthetic will be injected into your groin, or less commonly your arm, before a needle is inserted into your artery (see p88). You should feel slight pressure as the catheter is placed and moved up the aorta to your coronary arteries. You may feel fleeting chest pain when the dye is injected. This straightforward procedure takes about 20–30 minutes.

Q Will the cardiologist take a look at my heart function, too?

Yes, possibly. After examining the coronary arteries, the catheter may be advanced into the left ventricle and more dye injected. The same X-ray/movie sequence is performed and the cardiologist can then analyze the performance of the left ventricle and check the valves. If a picture of the heart muscle function is taken, you may feel a hot flash from head to toe, lasting about 20 seconds as the dye passes through your body.

VIEWING THE CORONARY ARTERIES

Heart specialists can determine the condition of the coronary arteries by using an imaging technique called angiography. The procedure produces a moving image called an angiogram that reveals whether the arteries are narrowed or even blocked.

The first part of the procedure involves inserting a fine, flexible tube called a catheter into an artery, most commonly in the thigh (below) but occasionally in the arm, and feeding it up the aorta so that the tip is in a coronary artery (below). As dye injected into the catheter fills the artery and its branching vessels, X-rays are taken. The catheter is moved to another coronary artery and the process repeated.

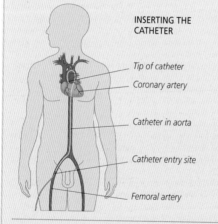

INSERTING THE CATHETER

Tip of catheter

Coronary artery

Catheter in aorta

Catheter entry site

Femoral artery

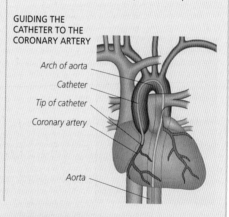

GUIDING THE CATHETER TO THE CORONARY ARTERY

Arch of aorta

Catheter

Tip of catheter

Coronary artery

Aorta

Coronary angiogram

Examination of a coronary angiogram (right) may reveal the arteries and blood vessels that are normal and healthy, and those that are narrowed or blocked. In this way, heart specialists can determine whether any abnormalities are severe enough to require treatment such as an angioplasty or stent, or surgery.

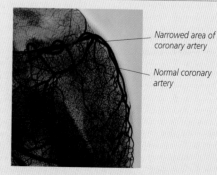

Narrowed area of coronary artery

Normal coronary artery

Q What is the main reason for having coronary angiography?

The main reason is because your doctor suspects that you have coronary artery disease. This may be because of anginal symptoms or because exercise testing revealed a significant abnormality – for example, your blood pressure fell or you had large areas of heart muscle at risk. The test identifies whether you need additional treatment such as medication, a catheter (percutaneous) intervention such as an angioplasty or stent, or bypass surgery.

Q Can angiography help with other heart-related problems?

Yes. Angiography can be used to check people who have some kind of unexplained chest pain. It can also help to test patients with valvular disease.

Q Are there other occasions when angiography is needed?

Yes. Angiography may be needed to evaluate an individual having other cardiac surgery – for example, a 67-year-old scheduled for valvular heart surgery – for silent coronary artery disease. Angiography may be part of an annual check-up following heart transplant, since transplanted hearts are prone to developing coronary artery disease.

Q Are there other technologies to evaluate coronary arteries?

Yes, there are several. First, intravascular sonography is an invasive technique that creates a cross-sectional view of the arteries and can detect mild blockages better than angiography. Second, a specialized scanning technique, known as (spiral) computed tomography (CT) coronary angiography, is non-invasive and can detect over 90 per cent of the coronary disease detected by angiography. Third, magnetic resonance angiography (MRA) provides imaging of the coronary arteries as well as the heart function and valve competence.

Blood tests

Q Can blood tests reliably foretell that cardiovascular disease will occur?

Yes. Although cardiovascular disorders have potentially many causes, there are certain predictive blood tests that can indicate if an individual is more likely than others to develop cardiovascular disease. Genetics and family history play a role in this likelihood. So do other risk factors such as a history of cigarette smoking, and obesity, hypertension, and diabetes.

Q What are the blood tests that have a predictive role?

An increased cholesterol level in the blood is the main predictive test. A total cholesterol in excess of 200mg/dL is an independent risk factor. The components that make up the bulk of the total cholesterol (LDL and HDL) are also independent risk factors (see pp38–39). However, it is important to realize that over half of the people with heart problems have normal cholesterol levels.

Q Does the presence of C-reactive protein help with diagnosis of cardiovascular disease?

Yes. The protein known as CRP is produced by the liver as part of an immune response to infection or inflammation. Its presence in the blood indicates that there is some inflammation in the body. Although it is not specific to heart disease, increased levels are associated with risk of coronary heart disease, sudden death, and peripheral arterial disease (see pp56–57). Therefore, a positive CRP blood test can contribute to a diagnosis of coronary artery disease.

Q Can raised levels of homocysteine also help with diagnosis?

Yes. When blood levels of the amino acid homocysteine are very elevated, they correspond to accelerated levels of cardiovascular disease. High homocysteine levels may also indicate an increased risk of stroke.

Q What is the most reliable indicator of a heart attack?

Two out of three criteria are necessary to establish the diagnosis of a heart attack (myocardial infarction, or MI). The first is symptoms of chest pain and the second criterion is an ECG that shows changes that are likely to indicate an acute MI. Third is a documented rise in the blood of certain enzymes (cardiac markers) that are released from damaged cardiac tissue. This is the most reliable indicator of a heart attack or cardiac injury. Around 15 per cent of those who sustain an MI have a "silent heart attack" – they don't complain of chest pain. Perhaps 25 per cent will not show any changes on an ECG. However, a damaged heart cell will *always* release cardiac markers.

Q What are these enzymes that are known as cardiac markers?

In the past, blood tests looked for two enzymes – lactic dehydrogenase (LDH) and creatine kinase (CK). However, these were not entirely specific to heart (myocardial) tissue, nor always reliably released with heart injury. They have been superseded by troponins.

Q When is the enzyme creatine kinase released?

Creatine kinase (CK) is detectable in the blood in those people who have sustained myocardial damage within four to eight hours after the event of a heart attack. It will remain elevated for two to three days. The CK test was the standard blood test for a heart attack, but is now frequently superseded by troponins.

Q How do the troponin enzymes compare with creatine kinase?

The level of troponins in the blood begins to rise within three hours after myocardial damage and remains elevated for nearly two weeks. Troponin enzymes are more sensitive than creatine kinase, and their levels rise earlier in the blood and remain elevated for longer. In clinical practice today, both enzymes are measured.

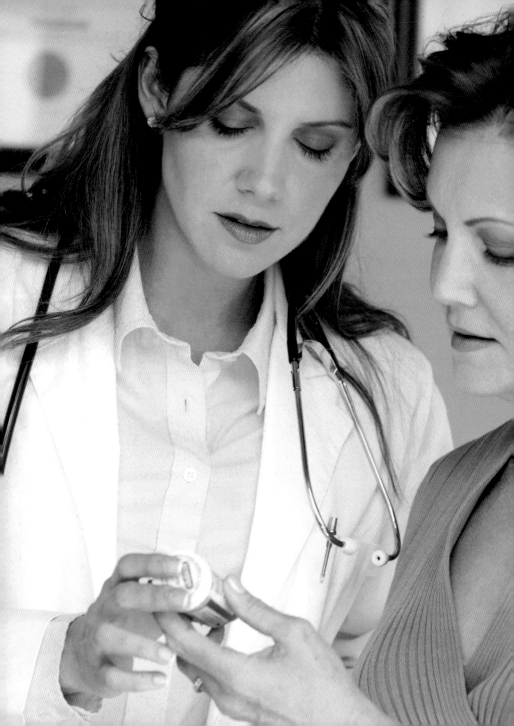

Treating heart disease

Early intervention is one of the watchwords in the treatment of heart diseases. The sooner a problem is detected the quicker it can be treated with either surgery or medication. Successful treatments have progressed with advances in surgical techniques, such as valve repair and replacement, and the discovery of new drugs that target specific problems, such as high blood pressure or elevated cholesterol.

Treating acute disorders

Q What is meant by the word "acute"?

In medical language the word "acute" refers to the fact that the disorder has come on suddenly, in contrast to "chronic", or long-standing, diseases. The response called for must also be acute. Speed is essential if a life is to be saved.

Q What action is needed in a heart attack?

A heart attack, or acute myocardial infarction, needs immediate medical attention because the heart rhythm may suddenly change, which can be fatal. Anyone afflicted with an acute heart attack should be treated promptly in a coronary care unit (CCU). There, steps can be taken to destroy the clot and thus "undo" the heart attack; arrhythmias (some of which are potentially fatal) can be effectively treated, and blood pressure alterations can be managed.

Q Can heart muscle be saved if it isn't damaged too much?

Yes. If prompt medical assessment indicates the acute attack or muscle damage is reversible, the patient is admitted to a CCU where "reperfusion" takes place. This procedure involves breaking up the blood clot, thereby re-establishing an adequate coronary flow. The threatened muscle, which would otherwise die, is once again provided with adequate oxygen and nutrients. Reperfusion can lead to a 25 per cent reduction in death that follows from heart attacks, but it can only be effective if accomplished within a small time frame – a maximum of four hours. If too much time elapses, the threatened heart muscle portion will perish. Clearly, the sooner reperfusion is undertaken the better.

Q Can aspirin help in this reperfusion process?

Yes. Aspirin should be given to every person who is suspected of coronary artery disease. Many believe that all people over the age of 40 should take aspirin daily. The action of aspirin is to prevent the platelets, which form part of the normal clotting process, from clumping together. Clots are most often the event that precedes a heart attack. They can fully block an artery that has been narrowed by cholesterol-laden plaques, and aspirin can prevent these clots from forming. Aspirin can lead to a 23 per cent reduction in deaths from heart attacks.

Q What can I do if someone's heart seems to have stopped?

Immediately call 999, unless there is an experienced medical person present to start CPR – cardiopulmonary resuscitation. CPR involves directly "thumping" the front of the mid-chest (the breastbone), then starting resuscitation, which includes both chest compression and mouth-to-mouth breathing.

Q What is DC cardioversion?

It involves giving the heart a brief electric shock to restart its beating. DC stands for "direct current," which is delivered with two "paddles" that are placed on the chest. The technique, known as defibrillation, may be used to treat ventricular tachycardia (see p64) or, more commonly, ventricular fibrillation. The latter is a rhythm that cannot support an adequate circulation and is a common cause of death following heart attacks. Treatment is essential, both to abolish the arrhythmia and – with the help of medication – to prevent the disorder from recurring (see p111). The most effective prevention today is the implantation of a small internal defibrillator (see pp112–13).

Q How is acute pulmonary oedema treated?

When the left ventricle is injured (acutely in a heart attack, or chronically with high blood pressure, valve disorders, or heart cell injury – cardiomyopathy), it fails to pump out the blood volume it receives from the left atrium. Blood then backs up through the passive left atrium into the lungs and fluid from the blood seeps into the lung cells (see p72), causing acute breathlessness. This process must be promptly reversed or it can be fatal. The aim of treatment is to rid the body of excess water by using diuretic drugs (see p117) and improving the function of the injured left ventricle with inotropic drugs (see p115).

Q What action is needed if my blood pressure suddenly becomes very high?

This is called an acute hypertensive crisis. The diastolic blood pressure rises to 130 or more. This is typically accompanied by some damage to the blood vessels – for example, to the retina of the eye (see p37). In more severe instances, the brain can be fatally affected. The treatment is to rapidly lower blood pressure with antihypertensives (see pp106–107), such as intravenous nitroglycerine or nitroprusside.

Q Can infective endocarditis be acute?

Yes. Acute endocarditis (see pp76–77) characteristically involves the right heart valves and is typically caused by a staphylococcus bacterium. It is most often seen in drug addicts. The bacteria enter the bloodstream from uncleansed skin, travel in the vein, and lodge on the right heart valves. Acute endocarditis can quickly destroy a heart valve, leading to cardiovascular collapse. Treatment calls for high concentrations of intravenous antibiotics for prolonged periods. Very often, valve replacement is required for survival (see pp118–21).

Treating coronary artery disease

Q How can my recently diagnosed coronary artery disease be treated?

Essentially, there are three choices – medical therapy with drugs alone, an angioplasty and stent (see p99), or coronary artery bypass (see p101). Medical reality, as defined by disease, and patient preference are both considered in the choice of therapy, and when symptoms are not relieved by medical therapy, a procedure becomes necessary.

Q How can I choose between surgery or angioplasty?

Coronary artery bypass graft (CABG) gives good short-term results, with excellent control of symptoms and improved survival. When multiple arteries have become critically narrowed, CABG is preferred. When only one or two vessels are involved, the choice is between medical therapy and angioplasty. You should make this complex decision with your doctor.

Q What does medical therapy involve?

If surgery is not required, your doctor may prescribe aspirin and a beta-blocker (see p107) to reduce the amount of work your heart does. Beta-blockers very effectively lower the death rate if taken following a heart attack. Your doctor may also prescribe an ACE inhibitor (ACE stands for angiotensin-converting enzyme). These drugs can prolong survival in people with coronary artery disease. A statin medication (see pp102–3) may be given to prevent new deposits in the coronary arteries from developing, and to reduce existing deposits.

Q What does angioplasty involve?

Angioplasty involves inserting a catheter with a balloon attached into an artery partially obstructed by plaque (see p99). This plaque is fractured and pressed up against the inner lining of the artery. A narrowed artery – often only one per cent of its original diameter – can be restored to almost 100 per cent and normal flow. This painless procedure is done in the cardiac catheterization laboratory using local anaesthesia. Inserting a stent usually prevents the arteries from closing. A stent coated with medications that induce an inflammatory response is even more effective. Medicated stents are now used with a year-long anticoagulation treatment to prevent late closure of the artery.

Q What is the advantage of an angioplasty?

Your recovery is prompt. You usually stay overnight in the hospital and you should be able to return to work in two to three days.

Q What is involved in major cardiac surgery?

In all cardiac surgery, such as coronary bypass surgery (see p101), the surgeon usually cuts through the breastbone (sternum) to fully expose the heart. To make the surgery easier, the heart is stopped and the circulation is maintained by a heart/lung pump, which is "primed" with blood. Transfused blood is used to replace further lost blood. The heart is still for less than an hour before it is restarted.

Q Is there a less invasive way to perform cardiac surgery?

Yes. New robotic surgery, in which the "surgeon" manipulates the "arms" of a robot machine, can accomplish the surgery through four small "holes". This is far less traumatic and recovery takes just a few days. At present this is only available in a few centres.

ANGIOPLASTY AND STENTS

Coronary arteries that are blocked or narrowed by fatty deposits can be widened by a procedure called angioplasty. This involves inflating a balloon at the site of the blockage and inserting a stent to help keep the artery open.

INFLATING A BALLOON

A guide wire is inserted into an artery (see angiography, p88) and fed to the affected coronary artery. The cardiologist feeds the deflated balloon catheter up the guide wire and positions it in the blockage. When the balloon is inflated the fatty deposit is compressed against the walls of the artery, restoring the blood supply.

Artery

Deflated balloon

Balloon is inflated

Balloon is withdrawn

Artery is stretched

Guide wire

Fatty deposit is compressed

INSERTING A STENT

Typically, a stent is positioned in the blockage to keep the artery open for a longer time. A stent is usually a tube composed of a fine wire mesh. It is a spring-like structure, and the cardiologist introduces the stent along the guide wire as before (see above), and places it in the area of the artery that has undergone angioplasty.

Deflated balloon and stent are inserted

Balloon is inflated

Balloon is withdrawn

Extended stent stays in place

Stent

Extended stent

Q Will I wake up from cardiac surgery attached to many tubes?

Yes, several. The most irksome is in your windpipe to facilitate and control breathing during the operation. One intravenous "line" allows you to receive drugs, while a second removes blood samples for tests. A "line" in an artery in your arm measures the pressure and oxygen content of your blood. A catheter in your bladder continually measures how much urine you are producing to show how well your cardiovascular system is doing. You may also have tubes inserted into the space around your lungs to help them re-expand after surgery.

Q When will the tubes be removed?

The breathing tube is usually removed on the morning following surgery, but you will be heavily sedated for that first day so you will barely notice the tube in your throat. Then, on successive days thereafter, you will have the remaining tubes removed. The chest tubes, for example, are usually removed after two to three days—and you are very relieved to be rid of them.

Q How long will I have to stay in the hospital?

Improvements in anaesthesia and pain control in recent years make it possible for most patients to go home within a week after this very major surgery. You should expect some restriction in your activities for a month or two after cardiac surgery.

Q What should I do and expect in this recovery period?

The cornerstone of your recovery is regular, progressive exercise. In the first week, start walking a little more each day. Avoid going out when it is too cold. Rest or nap when you need to during the day. See pp124–31 for more information about cardiac rehabilitation programmes and recovery from a heart attack and/or cardiac surgery.

CORONARY ARTERY BYPASS GRAFTS

One of the most important advances in heart surgery has been the invention of coronary bypass (CABG) operations. A blockage in a coronary artery is bypassed by grafting a blood vessel, either an artery or a vein, from another part of the body.

MAMMARY ARTERY

The two internal mammary arteries provide some of the best bypass grafts and may do better before they need to be replaced. At one end the graft originates as the mammary artery, while at the other end it is attached to the coronary artery beyond the blockage. As a result, the flow of oxygenated blood is restored to the part of the coronary circulation that previously had a restricted blood supply.

LEG VEINS

Where veins are used, the lengths of vein, usually 10–13cm (4–5in) long, are taken from a patient's leg. One end of a length of vein is attached to the aorta and the other end to the coronary artery. In the diagram, two blocked or damaged arteries (right) required two separate lengths of vein. Artery grafts do better than vein grafts because they are strong enough to withstand normal blood pressures.

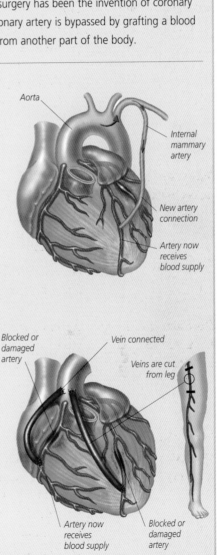

Cholesterol-lowering drugs

Q Who will benefit from treatment that lowers their cholesterol?

The most common cardiovascular disease is also the number one cause of mortality in the developed world and its incidence is directly related to the level of cholesterol in the blood. Everybody should be encouraged to have low cholesterol levels, but people who are at risk (see Chapter Two) should have regular checks in case they require treatment.

Q Who is at risk?

There are two groups in particular. First, patients who have known coronary artery disease have been shown to have a lesser risk of future cardiac events if their serum cholesterol is lowered. Second, those who are particularly at risk of developing the cholesterol-related diseases (diabetics as well as those with a family history of arteriosclerotic cardiovascular disease) should be particularly aware of their cholesterol levels. It is even suggested that men over the age of 35 and women over the age of 45 should "watch their cholesterol".

Q Is there an effective cholesterol-lowering drug?

Yes. Since cholesterol was identified as a reliable marker for the most common cardiovascular disease, the pharmaceutical industry has been searching for a drug that safely and effectively lowers serum cholesterol, while at the same time reduces the subsequent risk of related diseases. Since the 1980s, statins have been that class of drug. Statins inhibit a liver enzyme known as HMG CoA reductase, which is involved in making cholesterol. The consequence of inhibiting this enzyme is to induce removal of LDL cholesterol from the blood.

Q What is so good about statins?

Statins were a major breakthrough because they affect the metabolism of cholesterol in the body. They act on the liver to lower the dangerous LDL cholesterol in the bloodstream by between 20 and 60 per cent. Statins also lowered the death rate from cardiovascular diseases, but without increasing the death rate from other causes and they have very few unpleasant side-effects. The world has become a different place since the advent of these drugs.

Q Can drugs stop the absorption of cholesterol?

Yes. A drug called ezetimibe has been found to inhibit the absorption of cholesterol through the gastrointestinal tract and into the blood. Studies show that it lowers total serum cholesterol and also LDL cholesterol, particularly when combined with statins. However, studies have not yet shown that ezetimibe lowers the incidence of coronary artery disease, or the death rate from cardiovascular diseases. It seems that it is not enough to simply lower LDL cholesterol. In fact, it seems to depend on *how* the LDL cholesterol is lowered.

Q Are there other drugs to help lower cholesterol?

Other cholesterol-lowering drugs are available, but none are as effective or as safe as the statins (see p104). They include fibrates, which also help lower the serum levels of triglycerides, another type of fat in the blood. Bile acid sequestrants, also called resins or anion-exchange resins, are a group of drugs that stop bile acids from being absorbed into the blood from the gastrointestinal tract. These acids are released from the liver and gall bladder to help with the digestion of fats. The effect of preventing them from entering the blood is that cholesterol levels fall.

DRUGS TO TREAT HIGH FAT LEVELS

Your blood normally contains fats, such as cholesterol or triglycerides, but when they reach excessive levels in your blood your doctor may prescribe a drug that will help lower them. Such drugs do not solve the underlying problem so you will probably have to continue with your low-fat diet.

TYPE OF DRUG:	**STATINS**
Examples:	Atorvastatin, fluvastatin, pravastatin, rasuvastatin, simvastatin.
Uses:	To lower cholesterol (particularly LDL), and reduce your risk of heart disease.
How they work:	Statins work on the liver to increase your HDL levels and to reduce your LDL levels (see pp38–39). Statins are more effective than fibrates and resins.
Precautions:	If you are pregnant or breastfeeding, or if you drink a lot of alcohol or have liver disease, your doctor may not prescribe statins.
Side-effects:	Elevated liver enzymes in blood, muscle soreness, nausea, headaches, flatulence, constipation, diarrhoea.

TYPE OF DRUG:	**FIBRATES**
Examples:	Bezafibrate, ciprofibrate, fenofibrate, gemfibrozil.
Uses:	To lower the level of cholesterol and other fats called triglycerides.
How they work:	Fibrates (a) stimulate an enzyme that breaks down an essential component of cholesterol and (b) stimulate the liver to excrete sterol (another cholesterol component) into the bile.
Precautions:	Fibrates may affect the absorption of vitamins from the gut so you may need to take supplements (e.g. vitamins A, D, and K).
Side-effects:	Diarrhoea mainly. You may have indigestion or constipation.

TYPE OF DRUG:	**RESINS**
Examples:	Cholestyramine, colestipol, ispaghula.
Uses:	To lower the level of cholesterol and so reduce your risk of heart disease.
How they work:	Resins bind to bile acids from the liver, which prevents them being absorbed. As a result, the liver breaks down cholesterol to produce more bile acids.
Precautions:	Resins may affect the absorption of vitamins from the gut so you may need to take supplements (e.g. vitamins A, D, and K).
Side-effects:	Diarrhoea mainly. You may have indigestion or constipation.

Treating high blood pressure

Q Is there effective treatment for high blood pressure?

There are several classes of antihypertensive drugs that can control high blood pressure (hypertension) without severe side-effects (see pp106–7). In fact, most cases of high blood pressure can be controlled by one drug or a combination of drugs. And if there is good control, the risk of strokes, heart attacks, and kidney disease is substantially reduced.

Q What classes of drug are antihypertensives?

Many of them have daunting chemical names but their action occurs in a number of ways – by decreasing the volume of the blood (e.g. diuretics) and by relaxing the muscle in the walls of blood vessels (e.g. hydralazine, alpha-blockers, beta-blockers, calcium channel blockers, adrenergic inhibitors). Vasodilators relax blood vessel walls, causing the blood vessels to widen or dilate.

Q How are antihypertensive drugs prescribed?

Doctors prescribe them gradually over a period of time. They aim to lower blood pressure by 10/5 (systolic over diastolic – see pp36–37) for each prescription. Hurried or drastic treatment will lead to side-effects. Diuretics are usually recommended first, and may be followed by an ACE inhibitor or an angiotensin II receptor antagonist (see pp106–7). Then, a beta-blocker or a calcium channel inhibitor may be tried. Most patients require more than one drug to control blood pressure effectively, and it may take a little time to find the right combination.

DRUGS TO TREAT HIGH BLOOD PRESSURE

If you have been diagnosed with high blood pressure (hypertension) your doctor may try to establish if there is an underlying disorder that needs to be treated. If no cause can be found, then your doctor will recommend lifestyle changes – stopping smoking, weight reduction, exercise, low-salt diet, etc.– and probably prescribe one or a combination of antihypertensive drugs.

TYPE OF DRUG:	**DIURETICS**
Examples:	Bendroflumethiazide, indapamide, amiloride, triamterene, spironolactone, furosemide, bumetanide, hydrochlorothiazide.
How they work:	Diuretics act on the kidneys and cause them to remove more water than usual from the blood. This has the effect of reducing the volume of blood and lowering blood pressure (there also seems to be a blood-pressure-lowering effect over and beyond the diuretic effect).
Precautions:	Diabetics may experience problems because their blood sugar increases. Others may need potassium supplements. There is an increased risk of gout because uric acid levels in the blood increase when taking diuretics.
Side-effects:	Generally diuretics are very well tolerated, but confusion, weakness, and abnormal heart rhythms due to loss of potassium may occur.
TYPE OF DRUG:	**ACE INHIBITORS**
Examples:	Captopril, cilazapril, enalapril, fosinopril, imidapril, lisinopril, moexipril, perindopril, quinapril, ramipril, trandolapril.
How they work:	ACE (angiotensin-converting enzyme) is involved in the production of a chemical called angiotensin II (see below), which constricts blood vessels and raises blood pressure. ACE inhibitors block ACE and dilate blood vessels.
Precautions:	They are not appropriate when blood pressure is unstable because it may fall too low. They may not be suitable if you are pregnant or are taking diuretic tablets (see above). They may affect the kidneys.
Side-effects:	Dry hacking cough, flushing, dizziness, headaches, and fluid in the ankles.
TYPE OF DRUG:	**ANGIOTENSIN II RECEPTOR ANTAGONISTS**
Examples:	Losartan, valsartan, candesartan, eprosartan, telmisartan, irbesartan, olmesartan.
How they work:	They dilate the blood vessels and act similarly to ACE inhibitors.
Precautions:	They should be avoided in pregnancy and in the elderly.
Side-effects:	Similar to ACE inhibitors, but without the cough (a major advantage).

TYPE OF DRUG:	**BETA-BLOCKERS**
Examples:	Atenolol, betaxolol, bisoprolol, celiprolol, metoprolol, nebivalol (cardioselective beta-blockers); acebutolol, carvedilol, labetalol, nadolol, oxprenolol, pindolol, propranolol, sotalol, timolol (noncardioselective beta-blockers).
How they work:	Beta-blockers prevent the action of epinephrine, a hormone that causes blood vessels to narrow. They can be cardioselective by working directly on the heart or noncardioselective by working on the circulation as a whole.
Precautions:	They are not suitable if you have respiratory diseases such as asthma, or poor circulation in your legs and feet. Diabetics may receive less warning of a hypoglycaemic attack (dramatic fall in blood glucose). Never stop taking beta-blockers suddenly after long-term use.
Side-effects:	A general sense of weakness and depletion, breathing difficulties, cold hands, and raised blood glucose and blood fat levels.

TYPE OF DRUG:	**CALCIUM CHANNEL BLOCKERS**
Examples:	Amlodipine, diltiazem, felodopine, lacidipine, isradipine, lercandipine, nicardipine, nifedipine, verapamil.
How they work:	Calcium channel blockers prevent the movement of calcium in the muscle layer of blood vessels, causing them to dilate.
Precautions:	Not suitable if you have recently had a heart attack or have a slow heart rate.
Side-effects:	Minor side-effects include faintness, headaches, flushing of the face, swelling of the ankles, and dizziness when standing. Verapamil can cause constipation.

TYPE OF DRUG:	**ALPHA-BLOCKERS**
Examples:	Doxazosin, prazosin, terazosin.
How they work:	Alpha-blockers dilate the blood vessels by stopping the nerve impulses that cause them to constrict, and have weak antihypertensive properties.
Precautions:	Alcohol may enhance some of the side-effects.
Side-effects:	Nausea, drowsiness, headaches, blocked nose, and the risk of low blood pressure when standing up.

TYPE OF DRUG:	**ADRENERGIC INHIBITORS**
Examples:	Clonidine, methyldopa.
How they work:	Adrenergic inhibitors act on the brain's mechanism for controlling the diameter of blood vessels, which dilate as a result.
Precautions:	Reduced doses needed in the elderly, as with all medications.
Side-effects:	Drowsiness and headaches. Depression is a rare complication.

Treating angina

Q What drugs can I use to relieve the chest pain of an angina attack?

The main drug is nitroglycerine (GTN) or nitrate. It is available as a quick-acting tablet that you place under your tongue. Take it while you're sitting to avoid fainting as your blood pressure may fall. Slow-release forms of the drug are available as tablets and patches.

Q How does nitroglycerine work?

It relaxes the smooth muscle in the wall of the coronary arteries, which increases the flow of blood and reduces blood pressure. Most importantly, the chest pain is relieved. Nitroglycerine also dilates the arteries and veins throughout the body. In fact, it is more effective on veins, so less blood is returned to the heart. Consequently, the heart reduces its workload per beat and thus demand on the heart is also reduced.

Q Do antianginal drugs reduce coronary artery disease?

No. However, some of the antianginal drugs, such as beta-blockers and calcium channel blockers, that are regularly prescribed – but not to acutely relieve an episode of chest pain – may slow the progression of coronary artery disease. Beta-blockers slow the heart rate and reduce the force of the heart contraction per beat. They reduce the incidence of repeat heart attacks if given to people who have sustained them. Calcium channel blockers, also known as calcium antagonists, dilate the coronary arteries and are very helpful in some instances of angina. They block the entry of calcium into the heart cells, which leads to a less forceful contraction, less work for the heart, and thus less demand.

ANTIANGINAL DRUGS

If you have angina you will be familiar with the episodes of disabling chest pains that can result, often when you are exercising or doing a strenuous activity, but sometimes when you are just sitting still. In addition to assessing the lifestyle changes you need to make, your doctor will probably prescribe drugs that will relieve the attacks and reduce their frequency.

TYPE OF DRUG:	**NITRATES**
Examples:	GTN, isosorbide mononitrate, isosorbide dinitrate.
How they work:	Nitrates widen the coronary arteries and other blood vessels around the body. GTN can be administered as a spray or skin patch, or taken in tablet form.
Precautions:	Avoid using the erectile dysfunction drug sildenafil if you are taking nitrates.
Side-effects:	Low blood pressure. Occasionally liver or kidney disorders. Headaches, flushing, or dizziness when standing up. However, in general, GTN is very well tolerated.

TYPE OF DRUG:	**CALCIUM CHANNEL BLOCKERS**
Examples:	Verapamil, amlodipine, diltiazem, nicardipine, nifedipine.
How they work:	Calcium channel blockers prevent the movement of calcium in the muscle layer of blood vessels, causing them to dilate.
Precautions:	Calcium channel blockers are not suitable if you have recently had a heart attack. Some can lead to a slow heart rate.
Side-effects:	Uncommon side-effects include fainting, headaches, constipation, flushing of the face, dizziness when standing, and swelling of the ankles.

TYPE OF DRUG:	**BETA-BLOCKERS**
Examples:	Atenolol, bisoprolol, propranolol, metoprolol, nebivalol.
How they work:	Beta-blockers prevent the action of epinephrine, a hormone that causes blood vessels to narrow. They also cause heart rate slowing.
Precautions:	Beta-blockers are not suitable if you have respiratory diseases such as asthma, or poor circulation in your legs and feet. Diabetics may receive less warning of a hypoglycemic attack (dramatic fall in blood glucose). Never stop taking beta-blockers suddenly after long-term use. Some patients must stop beta blockers as they are overwhelmed by weakness and/or depletion.
Side-effects:	Breathing difficulties, cold hands, and raised blood glucose fat levels.

Treating arrhythmias

Q How are arrhythmias treated?

This depends on the type of arrhythmia. Some drugs control heart rate in rapid rate rhythm disturbances, while others abolish the rhythm disturbance and may prevent the recurrence of the arrhythmia. Implantable pacemakers can be used to increase the heart rate in slow rhythm disturbances. In surgery, ablation (see p113) can interrupt the electrical pathways that produce rapid beat rhythm disturbances and implantable defibrillators (see p113) can abort the potentially lethal arrhythmias arising in the ventricles.

Q What are the various anti-arrhythmic drugs?

Classes of antiarrhythmic drug are listed opposite. Some drugs, such as procainamide and quinidine, affect the way electrical impulses are conducted by blocking fast sodium channels. More effective, but potentially more dangerous drugs, such as amiodarone and sotalol, have a similar action, blocking potassium channels. They can be effective in preventing atrial fibrillation, paroxysmal atrial tachycardia, and some ventricular arrhythmias. Beta-blockers are effective in certain rapid rhythm disturbances. Calcium channel blockers are sometimes useful in treating rapid atrial arrhythmias.

Q What are the side-effects of anti-arrhythmic drugs?

Procainamide can cause connective tissues around the body to become inflamed. Amiodarone can lead to breathing difficulty, visual disturbance, and thyroid dysfunction. All antiarrhythmic drugs have the potential to cause more serious rhythm disturbances.

ANTIARRHYTHMIC DRUGS

Abnormal heart rhythms (arrhythmias) that seriously affect the beating of the heart may be caused by a birth defect, coronary artery disease and other forms of heart disease, an overactive thyroid gland, or stimulant drugs. After diagnosing the reason for the arrhythmia, your doctor may prescribe one of a number of drugs to bring the beating of your heart back to normal.

TYPE OF DRUG:	VARIOUS
Examples:	Procainamide, lidocaine, mexilitine, quinidine, propafenone, flecainide, digoxin, amiodarone, and sotalol.
How they work:	They affect conduction of electrical impulses in the heart. Some stabilize the rhythm in the ventricles (lignocaine, mexilitine). Others stabilize the rhythms in both the atria and ventricles (quinidine, propafenone, flecainide, amiodarone).
Precautions:	Some of the drugs may further disrupt the heart's rhythm in some circumstances. They may also be be toxic so a test dose may be required.
Side-effects:	Dizziness on standing up and breathlessness on exertion. There may also be mild nausea, visual disturbances, and more severe arrhythmias.

TYPE OF DRUG:	BETA-BLOCKERS
Examples:	Atenolol, propranolol, bisoprolol, nebivalol, metoprolol.
How they work:	Beta-blockers block the transmission of electrical signals to the heart.
Precautions:	Beta-blockers are not suitable if you have respiratory diseases such as asthma, or poor circulation in your legs and feet, or a predisposition to heart failure. Diabetics may receive less warning of a hypoglycaemic attack (dramatic fall in blood glucose). Never stop taking beta-blockers suddenly after long-term use.
Side-effects:	Breathing difficulties, weakness, a sense of depletion, cold hands, and raised blood glucose and fat levels.

TYPE OF DRUG:	CALCIUM CHANNEL BLOCKERS
Examples:	Verapamil, amlodipine, diltiazem, nicardipine, nifedipine.
How they work:	Calcium channel blockers prevent the movement of calcium in the muscle layer of blood vessels, causing them to dilate.
Precautions:	Calcium channel blockers are not suitable if you have recently had a heart attack. Some are contraindicated when your heart rate is slow.
Side-effects:	Minor side-effects include dizziness when standing, faintness, headaches, flushing of the face, and swelling of ankles. Verapamil can cause constipation.

Q How is sick sinus syndrome treated?

In sick sinus syndrome (see p61) the cardiologist will tailor the treatment to the characteristics of the rhythm disturbance. Typically, it involves the implantation of a pacemaker (see below) to correct the slow heart rate as well as medications to control the rapid rate arrhythmias.

Q Do premature atrial contractions require therapy?

Rarely. If they are particularly bothersome to the patient, then it is possible to treat them with medications, such as beta-blockers (see p111).

Q What is the most effective treatment for atrial flutter?

Atrial flutter (see p61) is optimally treated with DC cardioversion (see p95). Drugs, such as digitalis, calcium channel blockers, or the more risky but effective amiodarone, can return the rhythm to normal or slow the ventricular heart rate.

PACEMAKER FOR THE HEART

ARTIFICIAL PACEMAKERS

Artificial pacemakers are compact, battery-operated devices that take over initiation of the heartbeat. They are placed in people who have a slow heart beat. The device is implanted under the collarbone on the right side and connected to the heart. The pacemaker generates an electrical pulse every second or so. It also senses when the heart is beating and stops initiating the beat – so the heart and pacemaker only initiate a heart beat every second.

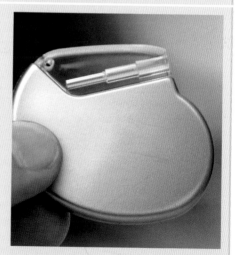

Q How is atrial fibrillation treated?

When atrial fibrillation (see p63) occurs for the first time or recurs but is not chronic, it can be treated with DC cardioversion (see p95). If not, it is treated with drugs to slow down the speed of electrical impulses and give the ventricles time to fill with blood. If A. fib persists beyond 24 hours, clots may form in the atria, so treatment includes an anticoagulant. Identifying the areas in the atria that initiate the fibrillation and removing them by using high-frequency waves – a procedure called ablation – can offer a potential cure.

Q Is it essential to treat supraventricular tachycardia?

Generally, supraventricular tachycardias (see p63) occur in otherwise fit people, but they can happen in patients with heart disease. Attacks of palpitations are often brief and require no treatment. If the rapid heart beat lasts beyond a few minutes, drugs such as digitalis, beta-blockers, or calcium channel blockers may be needed. Ablation (see above) can also be used if the attacks are troublesome and causative pathways can be identified.

Q How are ventricular premature contractions treated?

These contractions (see p63) are very common in the general population and may not need to be treated. In heart disease, they are potentially more significant and may require treatment with drugs.

Q How is an acute episode of ventricular tachycardia (VT) treated?

To abort a sustained episode of potentially fatal VT (see p64), either DC cardioversion (see p95) is performed or intravenous amiodarone or lignocaine given. Remedies to prevent further attacks are amiodarone, procainamide, or beta-blockers. A DC cardioversion device known as an automatic implantable cardioverter defibrillator (AICD) can be implanted like a pacemaker (see p112).

Myth "An early diagnosis can help your treatment to be successful"

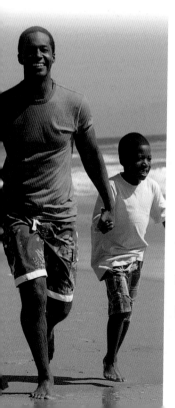

Truth This is true. Many heart diseases take a long time to materialize into symptoms that are problematic. For example, coronary artery disease begins with small cholesterol deposits that may take decades to produce symptoms. Even fit and healthy people may harbour some form of heart disease that can be detected in regular check-ups. As with many conditions, the sooner you are diagnosed the more likely it is that treatment will be successful.

Treating heart failure

Q My father has heart failure. Can drugs cure him?

No, but drugs can improve symptoms and prolong life expectancy. To treat heart failure (see pp71–75), the most effective drugs include a combination of diuretics, angiotensin II receptor antagonists, and beta-blockers. These are not always appropriate and others including inotropics may be used (see below). Since high blood pressure is the most common cause of a thickened heart muscle, good blood pressure control (see p105) can prevent, reduce, and even reverse the thickening. Your father should visit his doctor regularly, stick to his lifestyle modifications, and take his medication.

Q I'm on a course of diuretics. What are their effects?

Diuretics are medications that stimulate the kidneys to remove more water from the blood. In heart failure excess fluid may accumulate around the body. Fluid in the lungs causes breathlessness. So diuretics cause you to lose water, reduce the swelling in your ankles, and improve breathing. If your doctor prescribes fast-acting diuretics, such as furosemide and bumetanide, you will visit the bathroom several times after taking them. You may need to take potassium tablets to replace the potassium you lose (diuretics promote potassium loss).

Q My doctor has prescribed inotropic drugs. What do they do?

They are designed to improve the strength with which the heart's muscle contracts, increasing the cardiac output of blood. In other words, they increase the force of the heart so that it pumps more blood with each beat. The most common drug is digoxin, derived from the foxglove, which has been in use for more than 200 years.

Q My mother is taking ACE inhibitors but she has a terrible dry cough—is this avoidable?

Your mother is unlucky because ACE inhibitors are very good for people with heart failure since they improve the heart contraction and thus reduce fatigue and breathlessness, and even improve the ability to exercise. A few people do develop a cough as a side-effect, however, and the cough is more common in women for some reason. Your mother's doctor will check to see if her cough is caused by fluid in her lungs and, if it isn't, will probably prescribe an alternative medication, such as an angiotensin II receptor antagonist.

Q Can medical devices help treat heart failure?

Yes. There are devices that can improve symptoms and prolong survival in certain groups of patients with heart failure. The automatic implanted cardioverter defibrillator (AICD) helps to prevent life-threatening arrhythmias (see p113). The biventricular pacemaker is like a normal pacemaker (see p112) except that it has an extra lead to synchronize the contractions of the left and right ventricles. Mechanical "circulatory assist devices" can be installed in some patients with severe heart failure.

Q Can a biventricular pacemaker help my mother?

If your mother demonstrates delayed electrical activity of the heart, there is a 50 per cent chance that a biventricular pacemaker will improve her symptoms.

Q Are there surgical procedures that can help a failing heart?

Surgical procedures, including CABG (see p101), may help. Valve surgery (see pp118–121) can be necessary if the heart failure is caused by an abnormal valve (see pp67–70). For a few people who have advanced heart failure, a heart transplant or surgery to implant a heart pump, called a left ventricular assist device (LVAD), may be other options to consider.

SELECTED DRUGS TO TREAT HEART FAILURE

When the heart fails to pump efficiently, inadequate amounts of blood are circulated to the body and fluid collects in the lungs. Combinations of drugs remove excess fluid, improve the performance of the heart, reduce symptoms, and prolong survival.

TYPE OF DRUG:	**DIURETICS**
Examples:	Bumetanide, furosemide, torsemide, spironolactone, zaroxalyn.
How they work:	Diuretics cause the kidneys to excrete extra water, reducing the volume of blood in the circulatory system and surrounding tissues.
Precautions:	Diabetics should be mindful of increased blood sugar. Others may need potassium supplements. There is also an increased risk of gout.
Side-effects:	Confusion, weakness, abnormal heart rhythms due to low potassium.

TYPE OF DRUG:	**ACE INHIBITORS AND ANGIOTENSIN RECEPTOR ANTAGONISTS**
Examples:	Captopril, lisinopril, ramipril, enalapril, quinapril, losartan, valsartan, candesartan.
How they work:	Reduce the pressure the weakened heart pumps against; modulate harmful elevated hormones (see p.106); improve symptoms; and prolong survival.
Precautions:	Need to be used cautiously if your blood pressure is unstable as it may fall too low. They may not be suitable if you are pregnant. May affect the kidneys.
Side-effects:	See p.106.

TYPE OF DRUG:	**BETA BLOCKERS**
Examples:	Carvedilol, metoprolol, bisoprolol, bucindolol.
How they work:	Also modulate elevated hormones that cause worsening heart failure (see p.107); improve symptoms and prolong survival.
Precautions:	Need to be used cautiously if your blood pressure is unstable as it may fall too low; must be initiated gradually to avoid worsening heart failure.
Side-effects:	See p.107.

TYPE OF DRUG:	**DIGITALIS DERIVATIVES**
Examples:	Digoxin, digitoxin
How they work:	Derived from foxglove extract; used in heart failure for over 200 years. Improve force of contraction of the heart and slow heart rate in atrial fibrillation (see p.63).
Precautions:	Lower doses required in older patients and those with any kidney disease.
Side-effects:	Loss of appetite and nausea, an early sign of toxicity; may also give irregularities of heart rhythm.

Treating valve disorders

Q My husband has mitral regurgitation. Can the mitral valve be repaired?

Yes. Treatment for mitral regurgitation (see p67) focuses on relieving symptoms, then correcting the disorder by surgically repairing the mitral valve. Repair depends on where and how the valve is damaged. For example, cusps that malfunction can be stitched back into position, ruptured chordae tendinae can be repaired, and an injured papillary muscle can be repaired and reattached to the ventricular wall. This repair has many advantages compared to replacing the valve. There is less risk of mortality, no anticoagulation drugs are needed, and the repaired valve will work better than an artificial valve.

Q Can other valves be repaired or replaced?

Generally, yes. Aortic valves that are either stenosed or incompetent (see pp68–69) are usually replaced. Repairing an aortic valve is not a successful technique. See p120 for replacement of an aortic valve. Tricuspid valves (see p70) can be replaced when they are severely stenosed and repaired when they are incompetent. For the treatment of pulmonary stenosis and pulmonary regurgitation, see p70.

Q My daughter has mitral stenosis. What treatment can she expect?

Treatment for mitral stenosis (see p67 and p69), which is now less common, involves dealing with the consequences, then correcting the narrowed valve. Your daughter may need to restrict her salt and water intake, and to take diuretics (see p117). Her heart rate may also need to be controlled. To prevent infective endocarditis (see pp76–77) her doctor may prescribe antibiotics to combat bacteria that may invade the blood.

Q How will her narrowed mitral valve be corrected?

This has to be done surgically. The simplest way is to use an external device to widen the mitral valve and thus relieve symptoms. This can be done by inserting the device into an artery and feeding it through to the heart. Symptoms may recur in a few years and demand a more definitive procedure in which the defective mitral valve is replaced in open-heart surgery.

Q Will a repaired mitral valve ever need to be replaced?

Possibly. If the mitral valve has already been repaired and doesn't function properly, then a valve replacement will be needed. Rarely, the mitral valve is replaced when there is a deformity – for example, due to rheumatic heart disease. People who receive a replacement valve need to take anticoagulants for the rest of their lives.

Q What artificial valves do surgeons use in replacement surgery?

There are two basic types of artificial valve, which are also called prosthetic valves. These are mechanical and bioprosthetic valves. Mechanical valves are made from inert, sterile materials. Bioprosthetic valves are composed of tissue from human cadavers or from pigs or, more commonly, cows. Which type is used in a replacement operation is determined by the need for life-long anticoagulation or the predicted durability of the valve.

Q What are the various mechanical valves?

The original mechanical prosthetic valve, the Starr-Edwards ball cage valve, consisted of a ball in a coated cage. More widely used today are tilting disk valves. The St. Jude valve, for example, is small with two leaflets (cusps), and has a lower transvalvular gradient (less pressure decrease from flow through the valve), but also gives a lower cardiac output. More than 170,000 bileaflet valves are implanted each year in the world.

Q **What are the advantages and disadvantages of mechanical valves?**

The main advantage is durability – the valves function well for decades. There are three main disadvantages. First, they occupy a significant amount of the cross-sectional area of the valve opening, leading to an inherently narrowed valve. Second, they may cause the circulating red blood cells to be destroyed. Third, they cause blood clots to develop at an accelerated rate, so recipients have to take anticoagulants for life.

VALVE REPLACEMENT

A heart valve may need to be replaced if the symptoms of the valve disorder are affecting everyday life or if other surgical techniques do not work. Valve replacement involves open-heart surgery during which the heart's function is taken over by a bypass machine.

AORTIC VALVE REPLACEMENT

The most common valve to be replaced is the aortic valve between the left ventricle and the aorta. The surgeon makes a small incision in the aorta to access the diseased valve (right), which is removed. The surgeon leaves a ring of tissue in place, then stitches the replacement aortic valve to it. This new valve can be a mechanical or a tissue valve. The latter can come from either a donor or an animal heart, and has three cusps (leaflets) that open and close.

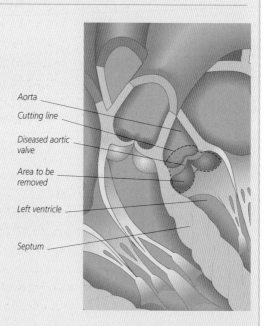

Aorta

Cutting line

Diseased aortic valve

Area to be removed

Left ventricle

Septum

Q What are the various bioprosthetic valves?

Bioprosthetic valves were originally salvaged from human cadavers and then suitably prepared to keep them from transmitting infection or triggering an immune response. However, they were impractical because the available supply did not meet the demand, and they were also fragile. The pig heart, which is similar in size to the human heart – and which functions in much the same manner – became a replacement source for prosthetic valves for decades. In recent years valves from cow hearts are more commonly used. Animal valves are also treated to prevent infection and rejection. Typically, they are stented (see p99) for better haemodynamics and ease of placement.

Q What are the advantages of animal valves?

The principal advantage of an animal valve is that the patient does not have to take anticoagulant drugs beyond the first few months when the risk of clots forming is high. At the end of this period the new valve becomes coated by the recipient's tissue and there is a lesser risk of clots. The flow characteristics (the gradient and cross-sectional area) of the animal valve are a bit better than the St. Jude mechanical valve (see p119).

Q What are the disadvantages of animal valves?

The most significant disadvantage is reduced durability. Animal valves tend to deteriorate over the years and so may need to be replaced. In some people, this begins in the fifth postoperative year. By the fifteenth postoperative year, approximately 50 per cent of animal valves must be replaced. Fortunately, this deterioration is gradual and can be monitored by echocardiography (see p84), so the valve replacement is a planned event and not a sudden, catastrophic episode.

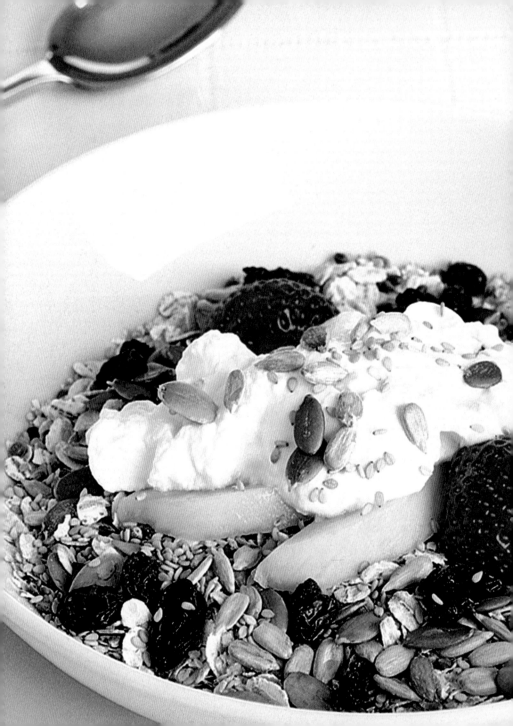

Living with coronary artery disease

If you have coronary artery disease, you first need to come to terms with your diagnosis. However, with good support and care you will soon be able to look to the future. You may have a heart disorder, but you should still be able to enjoy a rewarding and enjoyable life if you take care of your heart and tailor your lifestyle to your condition.

Recovering from a heart attack

Q What will happen to me during the first few days after a heart attack?

You will stay in a hospital for at least 48 hours to assess the degree of damage, and to monitor and treat arrhythmias. Techniques will be employed to reduce the severity of the heart attack. A member of the cardiac rehabilitation team will probably visit you to discuss your rehabilitation programme – this is a good opportunity to raise any concerns you may have.

Q Who are cardiac rehabilitation programmes for?

They are recommended for patients who have had a heart attack, but they can also be of great value for people with coronary artery disease who have not had a heart attack and for patients following heart surgery.

Q What is the purpose of the programmes?

The aim is to help you recover as quickly and fully as possible. The programme covers the key aspects of recovery from a heart attack or living with coronary artery disease. It will help you take the first important steps on the road to a healthier lifestyle that will keep your heart in the best condition it can be. It may also improve the prognosis after a heart attack.

Q Who will be responsible for looking after me?

Your cardiologist will continue to monitor your heart and general health as well as checking that your medication is working. Your family doctor will also play a key role in keeping an eye on your progress. They will be happy to give you information on your medication and to address any other concerns.

Q Who are the other members of my rehab team?

Other members of the rehab team will include physical therapists who will advise you on what exercise you need to do, counsellors who will focus on the emotional side of your recovery, and occupational therapists who will advise you on adapting your home life to your condition. These various healthcare specialists will provide you with a programme of activities, advice, and support, all suited to your individual needs, both physical and emotional.

Q What role can I play on this team?

You can play an active role in this programme – in fact, you will also be part of the team. The specialists will give you the information you need, but it will be up to you to follow the recommended programme so that you make the best recovery possible.

Q How long will the programme last?

The programme will aim to inform and support you through the stages following your heart attack – from the early days in the hospital, then at home, and right through to your long-term care. You will probably be able to start the exercise programme four to eight weeks after you had the heart attack. The programme may continue typically for up to 12 weeks in the UK, but longer in Europe and North America.

Q What will happen when I start the programme?

You'll start the programme in the first few days of your hospital stay. Initial measures include an assessment of your physical and emotional well-being. The adviser will also check for any risk factors for coronary artery disease that need to be addressed, such as smoking or obesity. You will be offered advice on appropriate levels of exercise, getting back to normal, returning to work, and the outlook for the future.

Q What will I learn about a healthy lifestyle?

You will receive information on all aspects of living healthily, but in particular the measures needed to look after your heart. Key topics include healthy eating (with cholesterol-lowering and weight-loss diets as necessary – see pp147–49), exercise (see pp153–55), and giving up smoking if you smoke (see pp151–52). Knowing why you need to make these changes should help to motivate you. You will also be given the advice you need on returning to work and driving.

Q Will exercise be a key feature in the programme?

Yes, definitely. Studies have shown that regular and appropriate exercise is a key component of successful cardiac rehabilitation. A physical therapist will assess your individual needs and work out an appropriate exercise programme for you. You may find that there are exercise classes in your area. If not, the physical therapist may recommend classes at the hospital.

Q Who will give me emotional support?

This is another key feature of cardiac rehabilitation and will be particularly important in the early days of your recovery. Counsellors and specialist cardiac nurses will give you support and encouragement. They also will advise you on keeping stress levels to a minimum (see pp158–59), which helps reduce the risk of further heart attacks. One-on-one counselling or group therapy may be recommended. Friends and loved ones will also play an important part in this, by helping you to come to terms with your condition and move forward. However, counselling may not be enough and a significant number of people who have heart attacks require medical treatment for depression (see pp160–61). Don't be afraid to seek help.

CARDIAC REHABILITATION PROGRAMMES

After a heart attack, and in cases of coronary artery disease, a programme of rehabilitation is recommended. It improves the prognosis following a heart attack and aims to set those affected on the right track for the healthiest life possible, both physically and emotionally.

A team of healthcare specialists help tailor the programme to suit your needs. They inform and support patients through the stages after a heart attack, from early days in the hospital and then at home, right through to long-term care.

Initial measures include an assessment of physical and emotional well-being. Patient support and information are crucial in these early days. The adviser will also check for any risk factors that you need to address, such as smoking, high cholesterol, or obesity.

You will need follow-up and support in the years ahead. Encouragement offered by loved ones and by the medical team is invaluable.

The components of the rehabilitation programme may include:

HEALTH EDUCATION Advice on how to live more healthily, appropriate levels of activity, and specific concerns such as returning to work and driving.

EXERCISE REGIME Regular exercise is key to successful cardiac rehabilitation. Advice from physical therapists and others ensure that the exercise is appropriate for you.

EMOTIONAL SUPPORT Counsellors and specialist nursing staff will give support in this key area. You will also receive advice on minimizing stress effectively.

CHANGES IN BEHAVIOUR In addition to exercising and managing stress, you will need to stop smoking, lose weight, and alter your diet to bring lipid levels under control. You will receive information on the role these changes play in protecting the heart from further damage.

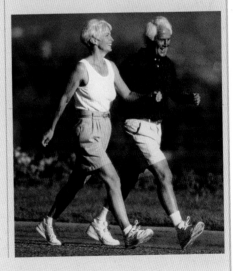

Myth "It is not possible to return to a normal life after a heart attack"

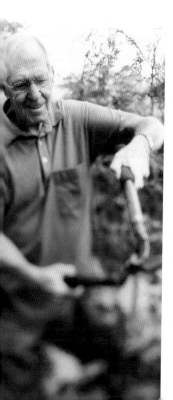

Truth Most people who have a heart attack are able to return to work and their usual activities, like sport, sex, and socializing, within a relatively short time. If your previous lifestyle was unhealthy, you can make changes that lead to a healthier life. This brings many rewards, not only in terms of keeping the heart as healthy as possible but also in making you feel fitter and more positive about having taken control.

Q What will happen once I get home from the hospital?

Leaving the comfort and reassurance of the nurses and doctors at the hospital can be frightening so try to make sure you have someone at home who will help with practical needs and give you the support that is so crucial in the early days. You should inform your family doctor about your condition. A cardiac specialist nurse may also visit you and, after a few weeks, you should be able to start the cardiac exercise programme, which will get you into training in a way that is appropriate to your condition. Don't be afraid to get in touch with your doctor or the cardiac team if you have any concerns or if you are feeling in need of support.

Q Will I need any special tests?

Your blood pressure will be checked routinely and your doctor may arrange regular blood tests to keep track of your blood cholesterol levels. You may have a treadmill exercise ECG test or other investigations, such as echocardiography (see pp84–85), that help to assess the condition of your heart following a heart attack.

Q What medication will I need?

You will be prescribed medications that help reduce the risk of another heart attack. You will need to continue to take these in the long term. You may take aspirin and/or clopidogrel, which will reduce the tendency of the blood to clot and make another blockage in a coronary artery less likely. It will also be necessary to take cholesterol-lowering medication. You may be prescribed an ACE inhibitor that will help your heart pump blood around the body if the heart muscle has been weakened by the attack. Beta-blockers are routinely prescribed as an effective preventive measure for a subsequent heart attack.

Q Why is maintaining my drug regime so important?

If you stop your medication you may increase the risks of developing further heart problems. If a particular drug is causing you problems, consult your doctor, who may suggest an alternative.

Q What do I need to know about my medication?

Having some understanding of your drugs will help you stick to your regime. If you are aware of the reason why you take each drug you will feel more motivated to take them. Ask your doctor about possible side-effects and what to do if they develop. Make sure you know when and how to take your medication – for example, should it be taken after or before meals? If you have concerns about your medication, speak to your doctor.

Q Are there any tips to help me take my medication regularly?

Taking various medications can be quite a challenge, but if you are organized you can stick to your schedule without much fuss. Try putting your medication out in the evening ready for the following day – divide it according to the timing of each dose. A special dosette box that lets you prepare your medication for the next week can help. It is a good idea to take your drugs at the same times each day and make it a part of your daily routine, like brushing your teeth.

Q What if I feel down and lack motivation?

Feeling low and anxious is only natural if you've had a heart attack. It is estimated that one in four people who have a heart attack suffer from depression. You feel you can't be bothered to make the recommended lifestyle changes. It is important to recognize when you need help – you may need counselling to help you through the early weeks or months. However, for clinical depression you may need medication (see pp160–61).

Q **What is the schedule for resuming normal activities?**

In the first days at home, you should take it easy. Wash and dress yourself every day to help feel more like your normal self and less like a patient. Light tasks such as making drinks and, later, cleaning up will also help ease you back into a normal routine. There is no absolute schedule for returning to work, driving, and other activities. However, you may find it helpful to seek certain guidelines from your doctor or cardiologist. (See also pp153–57.)

Q **When can I start driving again?**

The general rule is that you should not drive for about four weeks following a heart attack. After this time, you should check with your doctor to ensure that you have no medical problems that would prevent you from driving. If you have angina pains (see p55) when you are driving, you should consult your doctor and not drive again until your symptoms are brought under control.

Q **When can I go back to work?**

There are no general rules because the timing depends on various factors including your condition, whether your symptoms are now under control, your financial situation, and your job – if it involves heavy lifting, for example, or is very stressful. Talk to your doctor and your employer. It may be possible to return to light duties after six weeks or so – but longer if heavy lifting is involved. It's good to return gradually, increasing your hours over a number of weeks or months. Perhaps your employer can alter your role or the amount of work you do. Some workplaces offer an occupational health service that can give you advice on returning to the workplace. If you're nearing retirement age, you may feel this is the time to leave full employment.

The healthy heart lifestyle

Q What can I do to look after my heart?

If you have a history of coronary artery disease you will need to take a careful look at your lifestyle to ensure you are living as healthily as you can. Many of the changes described will not only help look after your heart, but should also make you feel healthier, happier, and more relaxed.

Q What do you mean by lifestyle?

Lifestyle is an umbrella word that is probably overused. It describes the way you live on a day-to-day basis – how you sleep, eat, work, have sex, and exercise, as well as the way you spend your leisure time and how you socialize. Lifestyle also refers to your pace of life. If your days are very busy and you have little spare time for relaxation, you may need to make changes to remedy this.

Q What changes do I need to make?

Several lifestyle measures will keep your circulatory system as healthy as it can be. If you are a smoker, giving up cigarettes is the single most important life change you can make. Making sure you eat healthily so your weight is appropriate and your cholesterol is kept within normal limits is also very important.

Q What about taking exercise?

Having a heart problem doesn't mean you can't exercise. In fact, your heart will benefit greatly from exercise, as will your general health and well-being. You will need to seek advice on the exercise that is appropriate for your condition and build up gradually until it becomes a regular part of your life.

Q What about stress? Dealing with your condition and coping with everyday life may make you feel stressed. Bear in mind that too much stress may cause your blood pressure to rise and this may affect your condition. You will need to take measures to learn to anticipate stressful situations and to deal with them when they arise. This will help you feel more relaxed as well as help you maintain your blood pressure at an acceptable level. Exercise, as well as taking the opportunity to relax every day, will help you in your stress management.

HEALTHY HABITS CHECKLIST

The following measures are important for keeping you healthy, whether you have a heart condition or not. Try to incorporate them into your everyday life. They will complement any medication you may be taking and help cut down your risks of developing further heart problems in the future.

Give up smoking – vital to reducing your risk of heart problems (see p151).

Maintain a healthy weight.

Eat a balanced diet that is low in salt, saturated fat, and sugar.

Keep your cholesterol within normal limits (see p148).

Do regular exercise as recommended by your doctor (see p153).

Look after your emotional health.

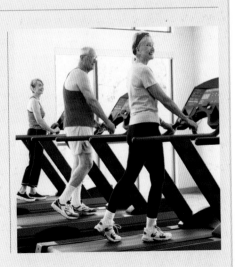

Finding out your healthy weight

Q How will my weight be assessed?

Weight is a more complex issue than simply standing on the scales. It is not only important to decide whether an individual is a healthy weight relative to his or her height, but also to consider build and the distribution of fat in the body. For this reason, in addition to considering your weight in relation to your height and body mass index (see pp136–37), your doctor may refer to the recommended waist measurements that are available for both men and women.

Q Why is my waist measured?

Over the years, doctors have recognized that a person's body shape is an important indicator in terms of heart disease risk. There are two main shapes – apple" and "pear" – although there are also thin shapes and a shape halfway between "apple" and "pear." The best way to assess these shapes is to measure the circumference of the person's waist and hips.

Q Which is the riskier shape?

The "apple" body shape develops as a result of the accumulation of fat around the waist. It is particularly linked with coronary artery disease and circulatory problems – even if the individual's body weight is normal. So the "apple" body shape is riskier, in contrast to the characteristic "pear" body shape, which is more healthy and tends to be found in women. Fat in the pear-shaped body is deposited and stored around the bottom, hips, and thighs.

Q How do I check my waist circumference?

To measure your waist circumference, place a tape measure around the middle of your body at the level that is halfway between the bottom of your ribs and the top of your hip bones. This will probably be equivalent to the level of your navel.

Q What is a normal waist circumference?

The waist circumference should not be greater than or equal to 94cm (37in) for men and 80cm (32in) for women. Above this level, you are likely to be at an increased risk of heart disease. Your risk will be greater if your waist measures more than 88cm (35in) if you are a woman and 102cm (40in) if you are a man.

Q Does the relationship between my waist and hips matter?

There is another measurement called the waist-to-hip ratio which can indicate a risk of heart disease. First, use the tape to measure the circumference of your hips and waist where they are widest. Then divide your waist size by your hip size. For example, if your waist size is 80cm (32in) and your hip size is 107cm (42in) then your hip-to-weight ratio is 0.76. This is a perfectly acceptable figure. But your risk of heart disease will increase if the waist-to-hip ratio reaches 0.95 or more for a man, or 0.85 or more for a woman.

Q Is it true that the frame size of my body could make a difference to finding out my healthy weight?

Yes, probably. There are three frame sizes – small, medium, and large – that take into account the variations in bone size, mass, and density, as well as muscle mass. Obviously, these three sizes are different for men and women. There are two ways of determining which frame size you are. The simplest is to measure the circumference of your wrist. Alternatively you can measure the breadth of your elbow (see p138).

Body mass index

In the 1950s and 1960s, when doctors and medical scientists needed a numerical way to determine whether a person was fat or thin, they turned to the body mass index (BMI) that had been developed over 100 years before by Belgian mathematician Alphonse Quetelet. It became a way of diagnosing people who were overweight or obese. However, the system is not very accurate and has a number of shortcomings – for example, it doesn't take into account a person's frame size, nor do these BMI values apply to children.

VALUES OF DIFFERENT BMI

Doctors still rely on BMI measurements to assess the risks associated with a person's weight and health, but also often use the measurement of waist circumference (see p135) and take into account the size of the person's body frame (see pp138–39).

The World Health Organization has published the following set of ranges for classifying the BMI:

A BMI of less than 18.5 means a person is underweight for their height.
A BMI of between 18.5 and 24.9 means weight is normal for height.
A BMI of between 25 and 29.9 means weight is above normal for height.
A BMI of between 30 and 39.9 means an individual is obese. If the BMI is over 40 the individual is very (morbidly) obese.

As a general rule, if your BMI is greater than 25, you need to take action to lose weight to bring down your risk of further heart problems and other serious conditions, such as diabetes (also a risk factor for heart disease) and some types of cancer. This becomes particularly urgent if your BMI is greater than 30.

However, there are some exceptions to the rule. For example, these BMI values apply to adults only; there are separate tables for children. If you are a pregnant woman or a breast-feeding mother, your BMI figure will not be accurate. People over the age of 60 start to lose weight in their bones so their BMI may not be reliable. Athletes and others with well-developed muscles also have inaccurate BMIs because muscle is heavier than fat.

YOUR BODY MASS INDEX

To calculate your personal body mass index, first weigh yourself and measure your height as accurately as possible. If you use the imperial system, convert to kilograms (weight in lbs x .45 = kg) and centimetres (height in inches x 2.54 = cm). Then use the following formula: divide your weight by your height and then divide the result by your height again.

In short, this formula is written as: BMI = weight/(height x height).
Alternatively, you can look at the BMI chart below to discover which range your body falls into – underweight, healthy weight, overweight, or obese. For example, a person who weighs 70kg (155lbs) and is 156cm (61.5in) tall would be classified as being overweight.

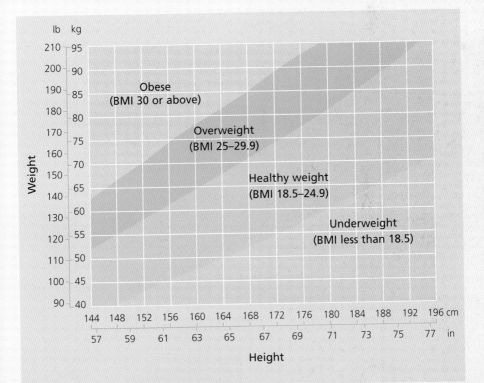

Obese
(BMI 30 or above)

Overweight
(BMI 25–29.9)

Healthy weight
(BMI 18.5–24.9)

Underweight
(BMI less than 18.5)

Weight

lb kg

210 — 95
200 — 90
190 — 85
180 — 80
170 — 75
160 — 70
150 — 65
140 — 60
130 — 60
120 — 55
110 — 50
100 — 45
90 — 40

Height
144 148 152 156 160 164 168 172 176 180 184 188 192 196 cm
57   59   61   63   65   67   69   71   73   75   77 in

Your healthy weight

One of the main drawbacks of using the BMI system to estimate what is your best body weight might be that it does not take into account the size of your frame. The tables on the right give the healthy weight ranges for three sizes of body frame – small, medium, and large – for women and men. To calculate your frame size you can either measure the circumference of your wrist or measure the width of your elbow (see below). Both are proportional to the size of your frame.

ELBOW MEASUREMENT

The following instructions will help you calculate the width of your elbow. Hold one arm out in front of you, with fingers straight and the palm facing upward, then bend your elbow until your forearm is vertical. You should be able to feel the two bones on each side of your elbow with your thumb and forefinger. Measure the distance between the two bones and refer to the chart below. Compare your height with your elbow measurement. If it is in the range shown, you are a medium frame. If it's less, your frame is small. If it's more, then your frame is large.

ELBOW MEASUREMENT FOR MEDIUM FRAME

Men	Elbow Measurement	Women	Elbow Measurement
157.5–160cm 5'2"–5'3"	6.3–7.3cm 2½ – 2⅞"	147–150cm 4'10"–4'11"	5.7–6.3cm 2¼ – 2½"
162.5–170cm 5'4"–5'7"	6.7–7.3cm 2⅝ – 2⅞"	152.5–160cm 5'0"–5'3"	5.7–6.3cm 2¼ – 2½"
172.7–180cm 5'8"–5'11"	7–7.5cm 2¾ – 3"	162.5–170cm 5'4"–5'7"	6–6.7cm 2⅜ – 2⅝"
183–190.5cm 6'0"–6'3"	7–7.9cm 2¾ – 3⅛"	172.7–180cm 5'8"–5'11"	6–6.7cm 2⅜ – 2⅝"
193cm 6'4"	7.3–8.3cm 2⅞ – 3¼"	183cm 6'0"	6.4–7cm 2½ – 2¾"

WOMEN

Height	Small Frame	Medium Frame	Large Frame
147cm 4'10"	46.2–50.3kg 102–111lbs	49.4–54.8kg 109–121lbs	53.5–59.3kg 118–131lbs
150cm 4'11"	46.7–51.2kg 103–113lbs	50.3–55.7kg 111–123lbs	54.4–60.7kg 120–134lbs
152.5cm 5'0"	47.1–52.1kg 104–115lbs	51.2–57.1kg 113–126lbs	55.3–62.1kg 122–137lbs
155cm 5'1"	48–53.5kg 106–118lbs	52.1–58.4kg 115–129lbs	56.6–63.4kg 125–140lbs
157.5cm 5'2"	48.9–54.8kg 108–121lbs	53.5–59.8kg 118–132lbs	58–64.8kg 128–143lbs
160cm 5'3"	50.3–56.2kg 111–124lbs	54.8–61.2kg 121–135lbs	59.3–66.6kg 131–147lbs
162.5cm 5'4"	51.7–57.5kg 114–127lbs	56.2–62.5kg 124–138lbs	60.7–68.4kg 134–151lbs
165cm 5'5"	53–58.9kg 117–130lbs	57.5–63.9kg 127–141lbs	62.1–70.2kg 137–155lbs
167.5cm 5'6"	54.4–60.2kg 120–133lbs	58.9–65.2kg 130–144lbs	63.4–72kg 140–159lbs
170cm 5'7"	55.7–61.6kg 123–136lbs	60.2–66.6kg 133–147lbs	64.8–73.8kg 143–163lbs
172.7cm 5'8"	57.1–63kg 126–139lbs	61.6–68kg 136–150lbs	66.1–75.7kg 146–167lbs
175.2cm 5'9"	58.4–64.3kg 129–142lbs	63–69.3kg 139–153lbs	67.5–77kg 149–170lbs
177.8cm 5'10"	59.8–65.2kg 132–145lbs	64.3–70.7kg 142–156lbs	68.9–78.4kg 152–173lbs
180cm 5'11"	61.2–67kg 135–148lbs	65.2–72kg 145–159lbs	70.2–79.7kg 155–176lbs
183cm 6'0"	62.5–68.4kg 138–151lbs	67–73.4kg 148–162lbs	71.6–81.1kg 158–179lbs

MEN

Height	Small Frame	Medium Frame	Large Frame
157.5cm 5'2"	58–60.7kg 128–134lbs	59.3–63.9kg 131–141lbs	62.5–68kg 138–150lbs
160cm 5'3"	58.9–61.6kg 130–136lbs	60.2–64.8kg 133–143lbs	63.4–69.3kg 140–153lbs
162.5cm 5'4"	59.8–62.5kg 132–138lbs	61.2–65.2kg 135–145lbs	64.3–70.7kg 142–146lbs
165cm 5'5"	60.7–63.4kg 134–140lbs	62.1–67kg 137–148lbs	65.2–72.5kg 144–160lbs
167.5cm 5'6"	61.6–64.3kg 136–142lbs	63–68.4kg 139–151lbs	66.1–74.3kg 146–164lbs
170cm 5'7"	62.5–65.2kg 138–145lbs	64.3–69.8kg 142–154lbs	67.5–76.1kg 149–168lbs
172.7cm 5'8"	63.4–67kg 140–148lbs	65.2–71.1kg 145–157lbs	68.9–77.9kg 152–172lbs
175.2cm 5'9"	64.3–68.4kg 142–151lbs	67–72.5kg 148–160lbs	70.2–79.7kg 155–176lbs
177.8cm 5'10"	65.2–69.8kg 144–154lbs	68.4–73.8kg 151–163lbs	71.6–81.6kg 158–180lbs
180cm 5'11"	66.1–71.1kg 146–157lbs	69.8–75.2kg 154–166lbs	72.9–83.3kg 161–184lbs
183cm 6'0"	67.5–72.5kg 149–160lbs	71.1–77kg 157–170lbs	74.3–85.2kg 164–188lbs
185.5cm 6'1"	68.9–74.3kg 152–164lbs	72.5–78.8kg 160–174lbs	76.1–87kg 168–192lbs
188cm 6'2"	70.2–76.1kg 155–168lbs	74.3–80.6kg 164–178lbs	77.9–89.2kg 172–197lbs
190.5cm 6'3"	71.6–77.9kg 158–172lbs	75.7–82.4kg 167–182lbs	79.7–91.5kg 176–202lbs
193cm 6'4"	73.4–79.7kg 162–176lbs	77.5–84.7kg 171–187lbs	82–93.8kg 181–207lbs

A healthy diet

Q What makes up a healthy diet?

The ideal is to eat a healthy balanced diet that offers all the nutrients the body needs while being low in fat, in particular saturated fat, sugar, and salt. By eating a balanced diet, you will not only be looking after your heart, but also ensuring that you feel as healthy and energized as possible.

Q Which are the healthiest carbohydrates?

Carbohydrates are found in vegetables, fruit, and grain-based foods, which are all key components of a healthy diet. Grain-based foods provide energy and come in two main types – complex carbohydrates, which are healthy, and simple carbohydrates, which are less so.

Q What are the benefits of complex carbohydrates?

Complex carbohydrates are the healthier option as they are rich in starch and fibre as well as many of the nutrients we need. They release energy slowly so they keep us going for longer and they are more satisfying. Sources of complex carbohydrates include wholewheat pasta, wholemeal bread, cereals, brown rice, oatmeal, cornbread, buckwheat noodles, and potatoes.

Q Why are simple carbohydrates less healthy?

Simple carbohydrates are processed and refined, so much of their nutrient value (vitamins, calcium, and other minerals), including their fibre content, has been lost in the manufacturing process. As a result of their lower fibre content, these carbohydrates are less filling and their energy release is rapid so that you will soon become hungry again. Sources include white pasta, white bread, cakes, and biscuits.

Q What about fruit and vegetables?

These are an essential part of a healthy diet, containing a wide variety of nutrients as well as being rich in fibre. Eating a variety of fruit and vegetables, at least five portions every day, is thought to reduce the risk of coronary artery disease. Even if you already have heart problems, this will help keep your heart as healthy as it can be while offering many other benefits to your general health. The fruit and vegetables can be fresh, frozen, dried, or canned. Leave the peel on when you can – it is a great source of fibre (see below).

Q What is a portion of a fruit or vegetable?

A portion is equivalent to about 80g (3oz) of a vegetable or fruit as eaten (drained if canned). Vegetable portions include 2 broccoli spears, 3 heaped tablespoons of fresh sliced carrot, 8 cauliflower florets, ½ a large courgette, a handful of mangetout, 3 tablespoons of frozen mixed vegetables, 3 heaped tablespoons of frozen peas, a corn on the cob. Examples of fruit portions: a medium apple, 3 whole dried apricots, ½ an avocado, 1 medium banana, 2 clementines, 4 heaped tablespoons of blackcurrants, ½ a grapefruit, a handful of grapes, 7 fresh strawberries (or 9 canned).

Q What are the benefits of fibre?

The two types of fibre have major benefits. Soluble fibre, found in beans and lentils, can help lower blood cholesterol levels. It is found in oats, too, so oatmeal makes a healthy, satisfying breakfast. Insoluble fibre, present in brown rice, wholemeal bread, wholegrain cereals, fruit, and vegetables, is not absorbed from the gut, but remains there and is then expelled from the body, helping keep it healthy and constipation-free. Fibre-rich foods help fill you up and reduce snacking.

A heart-healthy diet

There are various dietary measures that you can take to look after your heart. In addition to eating a healthy diet (see pp140–41) that contains a variety of foods and includes plenty of complex carbohydrates, you should remember the easy-to-follow rules to make sure your heart is in as good shape as it can be. For further information about diets that can help you lose weight, lower your cholesterol intake, or reduce the amount of salt you eat, see pp147–50.

KEEPING YOUR HEART IN GOOD SHAPE

EAT LOTS OF VEGETABLES AND FRUIT

Eating a wide variety of vegetables and fruit – and at least five portions every day – may help look after your heart.

EAT PLENTY OF FIBRE

Eat both soluble and insoluble fibre (see p141) – and remember, the soluble fibre found in beans and lentils can help reduce your blood cholesterol.

LIMIT YOUR FAT INTAKE

The total amount of fat in your diet should be limited. When you do eat fat, try to make sure it is mainly unsaturated fats (see p144). Cholesterol causes fatty deposits (called atheroma, or plaques) to form on the lining of the arteries (see pp38–39). Unsaturated fats lower the levels of the bad LDL cholesterol and help to look after your coronary arteries.

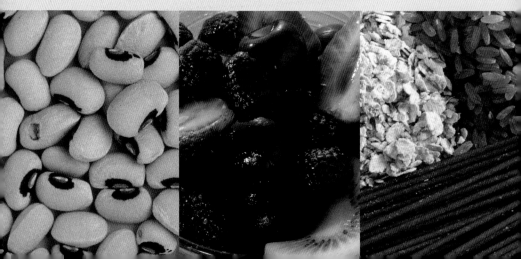

EAT MORE FISH

Fish is rich in protein, vitamins, and minerals. Oily fish, such as salmon, sardines, mackerel, and fresh tuna, also contain heart-healthy omega-3 fats. It is generally recommended that you eat fish at least twice a week and include two portions of oily fish. (One portion is about 140g/5oz.) Omega-3 fats are a type of polyunsaturated fat and are thought to protect the heart from coronary artery disease by lowering triglyceride levels and reducing the tendency of the blood to clot. The body can also produce omega-3 fats from walnut oil. Omega-3 oils may also improve the prognosis after a heart attack.

LIMIT YOUR SUGAR INTAKE

Sugar is high in calories and can contribute to you being overweight. Yet the calories in refined sugar are empty and have no nutritional benefit. Furthermore, the sugars found in sweets and cakes give a quick energy hit rather than the more sustained release of energy we receive from complex carbohydrates. As well as avoiding sugary foods, you should replace fizzy drinks with water and other healthier options.

LIMIT YOUR SALT INTAKE

High salt levels can contribute to high blood pressure, which is also an important risk factor for coronary artery disease and heart attacks. Therefore you should keep your salt intake to a minimum.

DRINK PLENTY OF WATER

As with a normal diet, drink about 6 to 8 glasses (1.2 litres) of water, or other fluids, every day to keep you from getting dehydrated. You will need more in warmer weather.

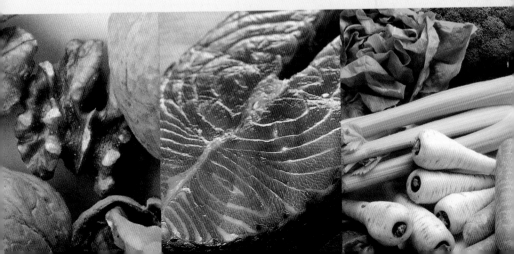

Q Why do I need protein?

You need proteins for essential functions, such as the repair of tissues. They are made of amino acids – the body produces some, but others (the "essential" amino acids) must be eaten. Proteins in animal-derived foods, such as fish, meat, dairy products, and eggs, are "complete" because they contain all the essential amino acids we need. Plant-derived foods, such as rice, lentils, and tofu, do not contain all the essential amino acids so you need to eat a variety of them.

Q Not all fats are bad, are they?

No. You need fats for the normal functioning of the body. It is nevertheless important to limit your fat intake to a reasonable amount and try to make sure that most of your intake comes from healthy fats.

Q Which fats are unhealthy?

Eating too much saturated, or unhealthy, fat raises cholesterol levels in the blood, increasing the risks of coronary artery disease. Saturated fat is found in fatty meat and sausages, hard cheese, and butter. Transfats are very unhealthy and may be found in cakes, biscuits, and pastries.

Q What are the healthy fats?

Unsaturated fats are found in many foods and are described as healthy due to their effects on blood cholesterol. Monounsaturated fats lower LDL cholesterol but not HDL (see p38) and are found in olive oil, walnut oil, and avocados. Some margarines are made from these fats. Polyunsaturated fats, such as omega-3 fats, are a vital part of the diet. They can lower the LDL cholesterol but also lower HDL cholesterol. They are found in sunflower oil, cornflower oil, and fish oil. They are also used in some margarines and spreads.

Q How much alcohol can I drink and still be healthy?

Drinking too much can contribute to an increase in weight and blood pressure. Excessive amounts of alcohol may also cause direct damage to the heart and can result in heart failure. Liver cirrhosis is another consequence of heavy drinking. The accepted intake (recommended by the Department of Health) is no more than 3–4 units of alcohol per day for men and 2–3 units per day for women. If you take prescribed medications, consult your doctor about how much alcohol it is safe to drink.

Q What counts as one drink?

When monitoring your alcohol intake, use these guidelines. Two units equal:

1 pint of ordinary strength lager or bitter.
A 175ml glass of wine.
One pub measure (25ml) of spirits.

Q What is the percentage alcohol by volume (abv)?

"Alcohol by volume" refers to the percentage of alcohol present in a particular drink. Ordinary strength wine is 12 per cent abv and ordinary strength beer is 3–4 per cent abv. However, always check bottle labels because many wines and beers are stronger than this.

Q What if I am drinking too much?

If you're stressed at the moment you may be drinking more than usual. Keep a record of how many drinks you have a day. If you are exceeding the recommended limit, you may need to seek help and support – perhaps in coping with the stress, but also to reduce your alcohol intake. If you're concerned you are drinking too much, there are support groups, telephone helplines, and online programmes that can help you.

Myth "Tea lowers the risk of a heart attack"

Truth It is hard to prove this one way or the other, but some research does seem to suggest that drinking tea can bring some beneficial protection. There is also evidence that drinking tea can benefit people who already have cardiovascular disease and who have had a heart attack.

Weight-loss diet

Q Why is my weight important?

If you are overweight it is important to bring your weight down to a healthy level. This will help bring your cholesterol down and may also lower your blood pressure and reduce your risk of diabetes, all of which are risk factors for coronary artery disease. If you already have heart disease, it is very important that you maintain a healthy weight. If you have angina, you may find your symptoms improve if you lose weight.

Q How shall I lose the weight?

The key to healthy, sustained weight loss is to lose the weight gradually at a rate of about 0.5–0.9kg (1–2lbs) per week. You will need to cut down your intake of food (the number of calories you eat) and combine that with an exercise programme that will burn up the calories and help you lose weight.

Q How can I change my diet to lose weight?

You may need to alter the content of your daily diet unless you're already eating healthily. Ask your doctor, cardiac nurse, or dietitian for advice. As a general rule, women can lose weight eating around 1,500 calories a day, men around 1,800. Don't count every calorie, just follow the simple rules for a weight-reducing diet.

Q What are these simple rules?

Eat plenty of complex carbohydrates. Eat fewer dairy products. Cut down your portion sizes of meat and fish if you need to. Reduce your fat intake. Limit your sugar intake. Include low-sugar and low-fat options when you can. Limit your alcohol intake – alcohol contains empty calories that offer no nutritional benefit.

Cholesterol-reducing diet

Q How do I know if my cholesterol is too high?

Your doctor will tell you after your blood tests. You should aim to have high HDL levels and low LDL levels in your blood (see p39). The normal limits are:
- a total cholesterol level under 200mg/dL.
- an LDL cholesterol level under 115mg/dL.
- an HDL cholesterol level above 40mg/dL.
- a triglyceride level under 180mg/dL.

Ask your doctor to explain all of these levels to you when you are discussing the results of your blood tests.

Q How can I cut down my cholesterol level?

You need to tackle the factors that may be contributing to it. These are: a diet high in saturated fat; a lack of exercise (this may raise bad LDL cholesterol levels and lower good HDL cholesterol levels); being overweight (this may raise your LDL levels and lower your HDL levels); and drinking more than the recommended limit of alcohol (see p145).

Q Will I need medication?

If your cholesterol level is high, medication may be prescribed to bring it down (see p104). This medication should be combined with a cholesterol-reducing diet, which will reduce the total amount of fat in your diet and ensure the fat you do eat is mainly unsaturated.

Q What about cholesterol-rich foods like eggs?

A few foods have a particularly high cholesterol content. These foods include eggs, liver, kidneys, and prawns. However, there is usually no need to cut these foods out of the diet altogether as long as you continue to eat a healthy low-fat diet.

Q How can fibre help?

Remember, soluble fibre can help lower cholesterol by limiting its absorption from the gut into the blood. This type of fibre is found in beans, legumes, and oatmeal. In addition, if you eat fibre-rich foods you will find they fill you up and make it easier to keep away from fatty treats such as chocolate.

Q Which are low-fat options?

Look for low-fat options with a total fat content of 3 g (0.1oz) or less per 100 g (3.5oz) and a saturated fat content of 1.5g (0.05oz) of saturates or less per 100g (3.5oz). Watch out for misleading labels – 0 per cent cholesterol doesn't mean other fat levels are low.

Q How much fat can I eat?

The body needs some fat, but do not get too many of the calories you eat and drink in the form of fat. As a guide, if you have 1,500 cals per day, your total fat per day should be around 57g (2oz), with saturated fat no more than 15g (0.5oz). For a 1,800 cal intake, the total fat would be about 68g (2.4oz) and the saturated fat level around 18g (0.6oz).

TOP TIPS FOR A HEALTHY LOW-FAT DIET

- Use small amounts of fat when cooking. Avoid frying and try grilling and steaming.
- If you're drinking full-fat milk, switch to skimmed or low-fat milk.
- Use low-fat spreads with unsaturated fats, not butter.
- Switch to low-fat yogurts and cheese.

- Stop eating red meat and replace it with fish and chicken.
- Avoid fatty gravy and sauces such as mayonnaise.
- Avoid pastries, chocolate, chips, biscuits, cakes, and other fatty snacks.
- Check labels for fat content and choose low-fat options.

Salt-restricted diet

Q How much salt can I eat?

The less salt you eat in your diet, the better. Salt can contribute to raised blood pressure, itself a risk factor for coronary artery disease (see pp36–37). Your daily intake of salt should be less than 6g (0.2oz).

Q How do I know if a food is high in salt?

Many of us are unaware of how salty many ready-made foods are. Always check the label for salt content (grams of salt per 100g/3.5oz). High salt content is classed as more than 1.5g (0.05oz) of salt per 100g/3.5oz (or 0.6g/0.02oz sodium). Low salt content is 0.3g/0.01oz of salt or less per 100g/3.5oz (or 0.1g/0.003oz sodium).

Q How can I cut down the salt in my diet?

Avoid ready-made and processed foods as much as you can. Eat homemade foods whenever possible – they are usually richer in nutrients and tastier too, even if you cut down on the salt you add during cooking.

Q What foods do I need to avoid?

Salty foods to avoid include crisps, savoury snacks, salted nuts, baked beans, some tinned vegetables, and many ready meals. You can buy some of these foods with reduced or no salt, e.g. baked beans and tinned sweetcorn. Check the labels – even cereals, bread, and biscuits – and remember the 6g/0.2oz-a-day limit.

Q How can I make food taste good without using salt?

Gradually cut down the salt in your cooking and rely on the food's natural flavour. You'll get used to eating less salt and will soon leave it out altogether. Instead of salt, try adding herbs, spices, lemon juice, or garlic, and use freshly ground pepper or white pepper at the table.

Giving up smoking

Q Why should I give up smoking?

Because it's the most important thing you can do to keep your heart in the best shape. Smoking contributes to the build-up of atheromata – fatty deposits on the lining of the coronary arteries and other arteries around the body, which causes narrowing of the arteries. In addition, smoking increases the heart rate and blood pressure, putting your heart under more strain.

Q I already have coronary artery disease. Will it make a difference?

Yes. A smoker can halve their chance of having a heart attack within the period of a year if they give up cigarettes. So it makes sense that, even if you already have coronary artery disease, you should give up to lessen your chance of having further problems.

Q How can I stop?

Smoking is an addiction, and a very powerful one, so giving up smoking will not be easy. Decide what day you are going to give up and stick to it. Cutting down gradually does not work. You will find it very difficult to cut out the last few altogether and will easily be tempted to start smoking more again. Nicotine and non-nicotine aids (see p152) can help.

Q What else is available?

Some smokers choose to visit complementary or alternative health practitioners to help them quit. Most often they visit acupuncturists and hypnotherapists. There is no scientific evidence to support the efficacy of these therapies, but they may help some people and may be worth a try. If you decide to follow this route, ensure your practitioner is fully registered.

STOP-SMOKING PRODUCTS

If you want to use a product, there are two main types – nicotine-containing aids and non-nicotine aids. These can be bought over the counter or acquired by prescription. In addition, you may wish to attend a smoking cessation clinic or call a helpline. Talking to others will give you the support you need and will help you stick to your decision.

NICOTINE-CONTAINING AIDS

Nicotine replacement therapy (NRT) aims to ease withdrawal from nicotine by releasing smaller amounts of nicotine into your system. NRT may double your chances of giving up. If you have a heart condition talk to your doctor first. NRT comes in a variety of forms:

Gum delivers the nicotine quickly and so can help keep cravings at bay. It may cause tingling and some irritation in the mouth, but this should settle with time. Nicotine gum is usually used for three months, chewing one piece per hour. It comes in two strengths – 2mg and 4mg.

Patches are stuck to the skin for 16 to 24 hours, releasing the nicotine slowly. You start with the highest strength, then gradually reduce it, usually over a period of two to three months.

Lozenges and tablets deliver about 2mg of nicotine, which is absorbed through the lining of the mouth.

Nasal sprays deliver nicotine very rapidly, which is good for cravings. They can be sprayed into each nostril up to 32 times a day, and are usually used for three months. They can irritate the nostrils, but this tends to settle after a few days.

Inhalators are like a cigarette holder, but with a nicotine-containing cartridge put into the holder. As in smoking, the user holds the inhalator and takes puffs from it. Nicotine is delivered to the throat, but not into the lungs.

NON-NICOTINE AIDS

Your doctor may prescribe the drug bupropion, which reduces cravings and withdrawal symptoms. A course lasts for two months and doubles your chance of quitting. You smoke cigarettes for the first week while the drug takes effect, then you stop altogether. You may have mild side-effects, such as headaches and a dry mouth, but these usually settle within a few weeks.

Exercise

Q What are the health benefits of exercise?

There are many benefits, such as increasing the levels of healthy HDL cholesterol, as well as helping lower blood pressure, thereby lowering the risk of developing coronary artery disease. Regular exercise helps reduce the tendency of the blood to clot and reduces the risk of heart attacks. It is also thought to improve the outlook for those who have had a heart attack. Exercise reduces the risk of strokes and of developing diabetes. In addition, it helps with losing and maintaining weight loss, while improving general well-being, and helping with stress management.

Q How much exercise should I be doing?

Ideally, you should aim to build up to doing some form of exercise every day and at least for 30 minutes five days a week. Your doctor will advise you on the amount and type of exercise that is suited to your condition and how to build your exercise levels up gradually.

Q How can I make sure I am exercising safely?

If you have had a heart attack or surgery for coronary artery disease, your cardiologist or cardiac rehabilitation nurse will advise you on the exercise that is right for you. If you are taking part in a cardiac rehabilitation programme, you will be given advice as part of this. Many hospitals and gyms run special programmes for individuals who have heart conditions. If you have angina, you will still need to take some form of exercise, but you should seek the advice of your doctor and build up your exercise levels gradually to avoid putting undue stress on your heart.

Q How will I know when to stop exercising?

Your body will usually tell you. If your exercise sessions are making you overtired or unduly short of breath, seek advice from your doctor or cardiac nurse on how to adjust your programme. If you become short of breath or feel tired, slow down or stop.

Q What should I do if the symptoms seem to be serious?

You should stop immediately and rest if you become aware of a rapid or irregular heart beat, have chest pain (as well as pain up into the neck and down the arm), feel lightheaded, dizzy, sick, or weak, or develop any other symptoms you are worried about. If the symptoms persist, seek medical advice right away.

Q What types of exercise should I do?

Aerobic exercise is recommended as being beneficial for the heart. It works the big muscles of the arms and legs, increasing their demand for blood and the workload of the heart and the lungs. Examples of aerobic exercise include walking, swimming, and dancing. You may be able to build up to more strenuous activities such as tennis and cycling later. Walking is an excellent starting point for your exercise regime because you can gradually build up your speed and the distance you can cover. Swimming is a good choice, particularly if you have back or joint problems. Dancing is also great exercise. It can be fun and you can do it at your own pace.

Q How do I ensure that I stick to my fitness regime?

It is important to find a form of exercise that you enjoy, so that it becomes a pleasure rather than a chore. You may enjoy it more if you join a club or do the exercise with friends. Exercise classes that suit those with heart problems may be available where you live. Find out at your health centre or local gym.

EXERCISE GUIDELINES

There are no specific exercise movements to work out the heart – you just need to do some regular aerobic exercise. Try to exercise with someone else because this will help you to stick to your fitness regime. Remember the following important guidelines:

Always follow the advice of your doctor or heart specialist.

Build up your exercise regime gradually. Do not over-exert yourself. As a rule, you should be able to continue talking while you exercise.

Don't lift weights or do any exercise that unduly strains groups of muscles.

Don't exercise straight after a meal – wait at least two hours.

Wear appropriate clothing and comfortable footwear.

Always warm up and do stretches before you start to exercise and remember to cool down at the end. Avoid doing your exercise in extremes of temperature.

If you use a GTN spray (see p109) or a similar medication for angina relief, take it with you when you exercise.

Continue to drink water throughout your exercise programme.

If you take a significant break in your exercise regime, make sure you build it up gradually again.

Don't exercise if you are feeling unwell or if you have an infectious illness or a raised temperature. Make sure you are free from any symptoms for a few days before you start to exercise again. Ask your doctor for advice if you are in doubt or have any concerns.

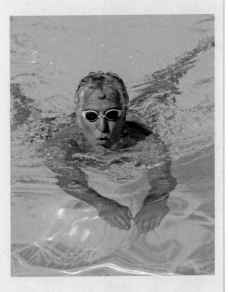

Myth "Viagra increases the risk of a heart attack"

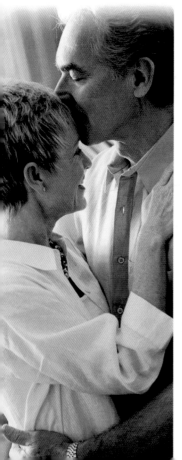

Truth When sildenafil, which is sold under the trade name Viagra, was first introduced there were reports of heart attacks and sudden death. Subsequent studies have suggested that, when they were not taking nitrates, patients with stable coronary artery disease could use sildenafil without the risk of heart attack or death. While these events indeed occur in patients with coronary artery disease, their incidence is no higher if they take sildenafil.

Sex and relationships

Q Can my partner and I have sex?

Having sex can raise the blood pressure and heart rate. However, if you can exercise, you should be able to have sex, too. Take things slowly. Listen to your body and don't over-exert yourself. If you've had a heart attack, you should be able to have sex again once you're better – maybe after a few weeks. Don't be afraid to talk about it with your doctor or rehabilitation nurse.

Q Are there any special measures?

You may need to change your approach to sex. You may be less energetic and your partner may need to take more of a leading role. Cuddling and touching will make you feel intimate again as well as helping you relax. Wait for at least two hours after a meal before having sex, and choose a warm place. Keep your GTN spray or other angina reliever medication at hand so you can treat any chest pain promptly if it develops.

Q I seem to have lost interest in sex. Is this normal?

Loss of sex drive is very common in people who are unwell or have long-term medical conditions. Men may have problems achieving or sustaining an erection. If you feel stressed about your heart condition, this may be a factor. In addition, some drugs for treating the heart and other disorders can cause erectile dysfunction.

Q What can I do?

Try not to worry and let your relationship resume naturally. Try to relax and spend time touching and holding each other. Speak to your doctor, not only for reassurance, but also to check for medications and medical conditions that can cause problems.

Coping with stress

Q Is stress a factor in heart disease?

We all experience stress at times. When we do, certain hormones are released to enable our body to cope (see p44). But if we are put under too much stress they may contribute to coronary artery disease. Undue stress also tends to make us increase other habits that are risk factors for heart disease, such as eating and smoking.

Q How do I know if I'm suffering from excessive stress?

Living with too much stress can present itself in many ways. Your moods may change as may the way you respond to those around you. You may also notice physical symptoms. It is important to deal with stress not only for the health of your heart, but also for your general well-being (see opposite).

Q What's the first thing I can do to lower my stress levels?

You can do many things to reduce stress and to make yourself more able to cope with stressful circumstances when you encounter them. First, identify the sources of stress in your life. Then develop ways to deal with them. A stress management course may help you do this.

Q What are the ways to deal with stress?

Do regular exercise to relieve stress and wind down. Eat healthily and reduce stimulants in your diet, such as coffee, which may contribute to anxiety and stress. Drink water as much as you can. Don't start unhealthy habits such as smoking or drinking alcohol excessively. Find time to relax and practise relaxation techniques. Talk to your doctor or cardiac rehabilitation nurse about stress management and counselling. Talk to friends and share your problems. Don't let concerns build up.

Q Is there a technique I can learn to relax? One good technique involves tensing and relaxing each area of the body in turn. Begin by lying flat on your back, with your arms relaxed beside you. Slowly take a few deep breaths. Start by tensing your toes, count slowly to three, then relax. Work up the body, tensing and then relaxing each muscle group. Continue to breathe slowly throughout. At the end of the exercise, lie with your eyes closed, breathing deeply before you slowly bring yourself up to a sitting position.

SYMPTOMS OF EXCESSIVE STRESS

If You have some of the following symptoms you may have a problem and need to take action to lower your levels of stress (see opposite page). Many of these symptoms are also features of anxiety and depression (see pp160–61).

- Feeling anxious and on edge.
- Being tearful.
- Experiencing odd aches and pains.
- Smoking/drinking more than usual.
- Working excessively.
- Being irritable.
- Feeling unable to cope with the practicalities of everyday life.
- Feeling more indecisive than usual.
- Having difficulty concentrating.
- Experiencing tension headaches.
- Having problems sleeping, such as difficulty falling asleep or waking early.
- Having a reduced appetite.

- Being under excessive stress may cause you to feel run down and generally lacking in energy.

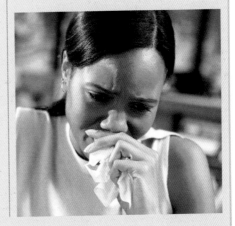

Dealing with depression

Q How do I know if I'm depressed?

Depression may come on for no apparent reason, but in many cases it will be triggered by a life event, such as being diagnosed with an illness. If you have a heart condition and are feeling low, there's a good chance you may be depressed. Depression is thought to affect around one in four people after a heart attack. If your low mood persists and you have other symptoms of depression, you should seek help right away.

Q What are the symptoms of depression?

Depression can cause various symptoms. These include feeling low (often worse in the morning), frequent tearfulness, irritability, an inability to cope, reduced self-esteem, feeling guilty, loss of interest in things, not enjoying activities as you used to, feeling everything is pointless, poor concentration, change of appetite, change of weight, poor memory, low energy levels and feeling tired, decreased sex drive, and sleep problems. Anxiety often goes hand-in-hand with depression.

Q What steps should I take to deal with my depression?

First, remember you are not alone. You are joining millions of people receiving treatment for depression. In fact, depression affects almost 10 per cent of the population, or six million Britons, in a given year. The important thing is to recognize you have a problem and to seek help and support. Depression is not something that can simply be brushed aside, but there are ways to get better and feel like yourself again. Talk to your partner or a friend for support, seek advice from your doctor, and think about joining a support group.

Q What is my doctor likely to do?

Your doctor will talk to you about your symptoms before recommending an approach that is right for you. If your depressive symptoms persist and are causing problems in your daily life, your doctor may suggest an antidepressant. These drugs act on chemicals in the brain with the aim of lifting the symptoms. Their effects may be noticed after a few weeks. Some of these drugs also relieve anxiety. Psychotherapy or counselling may help you learn to accept your heart condition and take a more positive approach to your life. Sometimes, this will be all that is needed to help lift the depression.

Q What drugs are used to treat depression?

Many antidepressants are available for individuals with heart problems. Your doctor may need to change your medication until you are taking an antidepressant that is right for you, both in terms of symptom relief and side-effects. The latter can be unwanted or beneficial, such as helping with poor sleep. Your doctor will probably advise you to continue your medication even if your symptoms are resolved. The idea is to make sure you that are well established on a more positive path before you stop taking the drug.

Q What can I do to relieve my depression?

If you're very low you will find it hard to take steps to feel happier. However, with the help of your doctor and possibly counselling you should start to feel better. You can now take measures yourself that will complement your medical treatment. Exercise, for example, will make you feel happier, thanks to mood-elevating chemicals released in the brain. Following your own interests and meeting up with friends may also help give you the confidence you need to return to a happier life.

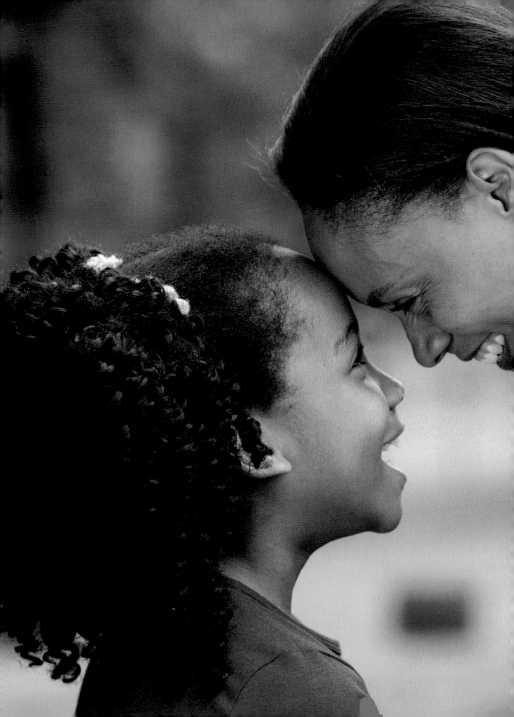

Special groups

It comes as no surprise that heart disease affects some groups of people more than others – for example, we know that smokers are affected much more than non-smokers, but they can reduce their risk by changing their lifestyle. However, some groups, such as the elderly, children, women, diabetics, and people who are obese, can be looked upon as special because they may have problems that are unique and cannot be avoided.

Heart problems in old age

Q Will my heart change as I get older?

Yes. Even a healthy heart may undergo gradual changes as a normal part of the ageing process. Heart muscle is not as strong as it was in your youth and may not be able to pump blood around the body as efficiently as it once did. Furthermore, your heart may not respond as well to epinephrine – the chemical that increases both the heart rate and the strength of heart-muscle contractions – to meet the body's needs during exercise.

Q Which cardiovascular conditions tend to occur as we get older?

As we get older we are more likely to develop heart problems, in particular coronary artery disease. By the age of 80, as many as one in five people have coronary artery disease that causes symptoms. Heart rhythm disorders and certain heart valve conditions, such as narrowing or stiffening of the aortic valve (see p68) are also common. So, too, is heart failure, where the heart muscle contractions are impaired (see pp71–75).

Q Can I expect high blood pressure to develop as I age?

Yes. With time the elasticity of blood vessels lessens, making high blood pressure increasingly likely – 80 per cent of people over 80 are affected. This brings an increased risk of strokes, kidney disease, and coronary artery disease. Have your blood pressure checked regularly – at least annually – and more often if problems are identified. With time high blood pressure may also lead to enlargement of the left ventricle and thickening of its walls as it tries to pump blood through vessels in which the pressure is high. This condition, known as left ventricular hypertrophy, may lead to heart failure.

Q I am a 75-year-old woman with raised blood pressure. How can it be treated?

If your blood pressure is only slightly raised and you are otherwise well, lifestyle measures may bring it down to a satisfactory level. These include stopping smoking and reducing weight if necessary, and doing appropriate exercise. In this way your blood pressure will be treated and important risk factors for coronary artery disease addressed. However, drug treatment is often needed, too. You will need check-ups to monitor blood pressure and detect any adverse effects caused by drugs.

Q I'm not that fit so will I be able to do the exercise?

Elderly people may be less able to follow the exercise programmes recommended for looking after a heart that is affected by coronary artery disease. However, you should be able to do some degree of exercise. Ask your doctor for advice about exercise that is appropriate to your age and physical fitness levels.

Q How is coronary artery disease treated in the elderly?

Drug treatments will often be the mainstay of treatment (see p97). Coronary angioplasty and coronary artery bypass grafting may also be considered (see pp98–101). However, elderly people may be put at increased risk by these procedures and sometimes other conditions or general ill health will mean doctors advise against them.

Q Can the medication cause me problems?

The changes in how the body functions with increasing age and breaks down substances such as drugs may make the elderly more prone to side-effects. For example, certain drugs for treating high blood pressure (see p106) and angina (see p109) may cause dizziness. Sometimes the doses need to be lower than in younger people or a drug may need to be changed. It may take the specialist some time to find the right combination of drugs for you.

Heart problems in children

Q What sort of heart problems can be present at birth?

The most common problem is a ventricular septal defect in which there is a hole on the septum, the wall that separates the two ventricles of the heart. Atrial septal defects can also occur. Sometimes the ductus arteriosus (see p31) remains open when it should close after birth. There could also be valve stenosis (see pp67–69).

Q What causes these heart abnormalities?

The normal development of the heart (see pp29–31) can be interrupted at any stage during pregnancy and shortly after birth. Causes can include problems with the baby's chromosomes, or a mother having rubella or taking certain drugs during pregnancy.

Q What kind of symptoms do the abnormalities cause?

This depends on the abnormality. Problems may appear in infancy, childhood, or even adulthood. Children may have central cyanosis, or blueness of the tongue and lips, due to low levels of oxygen in the blood. They may be short of breath if their heart fails to pump effectively. Some children do not grow or put on weight normally.

Q How will I know if my baby has one of these conditions?

Your baby's doctor may hear heart murmurs – often the first sign of a problem – at a routine check-up in the first year. They aren't always a cause for concern. Subsequent tests may include a chest X-ray, an ECG (see p82), or an echocardiogram (see p84). Increasingly, abnormalities are being diagnosed during pregnancy, often during the routine ultrasound scan at around 18–20 weeks, and with modern technological advances, it may be possible to operate on these babies in utero to correct the defects.

Q How will my baby's heart problem be treated?

After making the diagnosis the paediatric cardiologist will recommend treatment. Some conditions, such as small ventricular septal defects, may resolve on their own so the doctor will monitor the situation. In other cases, one or more operations can correct the structural problems. Some conditions can be treated without surgery. For example, an open ductus arteriosus can be closed at the age of about one with a special device introduced via a cardiac catheter (a fine tube that is inserted into an artery and guided to the heart). There may be a need for medication – for example, to treat heart failure caused by a large ventricular septal defect.

Q How do drug treatments differ for children?

Children need smaller doses than adults and these are calculated according to body weight. Some medications cannot be used in children so paediatric cardiologists carefully select the appropriate drug based on their experience and knowledge of the particular condition.

Q What heart conditions can develop during childhood?

Congenital heart problems are the most common heart disorders in childhood. Children with congenital heart disease are at particular risk of infections of the heart, either of the heart lining, including that covering the heart valves, (see infective endocarditis, pp76–77) or the heart muscle (myocarditis). Good dental hygiene and antibiotics before dental treatment and some operations are recommended to minimize the risk. Treatment usually requires a long course of antibiotics. Viral myocarditis can result in enlargement and weakening of the heart (cardiomyopathy). This condition is treated with drugs and, in some cases, a heart transplant may be needed.

Myth "HRT protects women against heart disease"

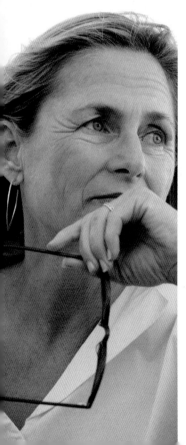

Truth Recent scientific studies have suggested that, contrary to the opinion that was popular throughout the 1980s and 1990s, hormone replacement therapy (HRT) does not provide middle-aged and elderly women with any protection against coronary artery diseases, such as angina and heart attacks. In fact, taking HRT may actually be associated with an increased risk of developing these conditions.

Heart problems in women

Q What special factors make women at risk of heart disease?

Around the time of menopause, levels of the female hormones, such as oestrogen, that offer protection against coronary artery disease dwindle. During pregnancy, the demands placed upon the heart and circulation are increased to meet the needs of the growing foetus, so problems may develop in around one in 100 pregnancies.

Q Does taking the contraceptive pill make me prone to heart attacks?

Not unless you smoke. The combined oral contraceptive pill, which contains oestrogen and progesterone-type hormones, is not associated with an increased risk of heart attacks in most women. However, the risk is increased for women who smoke. The tendency of the blood to clot may be increased in smokers who take the pill. This also puts these women at increased risk of a deep vein thrombosis, where a clot forms in a leg vein and may then travel to the lung and cause a pulmonary embolus. The combined pill may occasionally cause a rise in blood pressure, so this needs to be monitored.

Q Can I develop a heart disorder during pregnancy?

Yes, but most disorders are caused by pre-existing diseases. Women who have heart problems or high blood pressure should talk to a cardiologist and an obstetrician when they are planning a pregnancy. Women with congenital heart disorders may be at increased risk of having a baby with a heart disorder. If the heart condition is serious, a woman may be advised against pregnancy altogether.

Q What if I get palpitations during pregnancy?

Your doctor may detect a disturbance in the normal heart rhythm (an arrhythmia) during pregnancy and this may be associated with symptoms such as dizziness or palpitations. In some cases, arrhythmias found in pregnancy are associated with an underlying heart disorder, but in the majority of cases they will cause no symptoms and require no treatment.

Q What happens if I get high blood pressure during pregnancy?

This occurs in up to 10 per cent of women during pregnancy. If you develop a condition known as pre-eclampsia, with symptoms of high blood pressure, ankle swelling, and protein in the urine, you will need careful monitoring because of the danger of developing eclampsia, a life-threatening condition in which the blood pressure rises to very high levels. If the blood pressure is not brought under control, convulsions may occur. The onset of eclampsia may be heralded by headaches, visual disturbances, and abdominal pain.

Q Do many women get coronary artery disease in middle age and beyond?

This used to be considered a condition that mainly affected men. However, many women suffer with angina and heart attacks, too, particularly after the age of 50. Before the menopause, women may be protected from these diseases by female hormones, such as oestrogen. After menopause, these hormone levels dwindle and coronary artery disease becomes more of a problem.

Q I'm a post-menopausal woman, taking HRT. Can it cause me problems?

Yes. It might slightly increase your risk of coronary artery disease and also, for the first year of taking HRT, deep vein thrombosis. There is slightly more chance of getting breast cancer. There can be side-effects, too. You need to discuss these issues with your doctor.

Heart problems in diabetics

Q I am a diabetic. Can my illness affect my heart?

Yes. High blood sugar levels can increase the risk of fatty deposits developing on the lining of your arteries, including coronary arteries. High blood pressure is also more common in diabetics and diabetes can affect cardiac muscle, making heart failure more likely. In addition, diabetes can affect nerves such as those carrying sensations from your heart to your brain. This could mean that you might not experience the typical symptoms of angina. Therefore, you may not recognize you have a heart problem and this can delay diagnosis and treatment.

Q Are there any special risks that I should know about?

Yes. Having diabetes means that you are at an increased risk of conditions such as coronary artery disease and peripheral vascular disease. Women with diabetes are up to five times more likely to develop coronary artery disease, and men are up to four times more likely to develop the condition.

Q Will I need special monitoring?

Yes. Your blood sugar levels must be well controlled because the more stable your blood sugar, the less likely it is that heart disease will develop. At check-ups your doctor will look for signs of heart and vascular disease, as well as for other complications of diabetes. Your blood pressure must be checked regularly – your target is usually around 130/80. Your doctor will also check your weight and run a series of blood tests to check your blood sugar control, and your cholesterol and triglyceride levels.

Q What can I do to reduce my chances of developing heart problems?

There are many important lifestyle measures that can complement the actions of the drugs your doctor will prescribe for your diabetes and for lowering your other risk factors for coronary artery disease. This means exercising, not smoking, and eating a healthy diet to keep your weight, cholesterol, and triglyceride levels within the recommended limits (see Chapter Six). Bring your stress down to acceptable levels, too, and take time to relax as often as possible (see pp158–59).

Q How will exercise help me?

Exercise is one of the key things you can do to help reduce your increased risk of coronary artery disease. If you already have heart disease, you should still exercise to reduce your risk of further problems. Seek expert medical advice on the levels and type of exercise that are safe for you. Remember that you may need to alter your diabetes medication to keep your blood sugar levels within the appropriate range. Exercising regularly may reduce your diabetes medication requirements.

Q Will my heart medication be different because I have diabetes?

No. Your doctor may prescribe daily aspirin to reduce the tendency of the blood to clot and so possibly reduce the risk of a heart attack. You will probably need lipid-lowering drugs to bring your cholesterol and triglyceride levels under control (see pp102–103) and drugs to reduce high blood pressure (see pp106–107). As for people without diabetes, your doctor may recommend angioplasty to widen narrowed coronary arteries (see p99) or an operation to bypass them (see p100). If you have a heart attack, your anti-diabetic medication may need to be altered afterwards to ensure that your blood sugar control is as good as it can be.

Heart problems and obesity

Q I think I may be obese. What can I do to avoid heart problems?

First, find out if you really are obese by calculating your body mass index (see pp136–37), then calculate what your healthy weight should be (see pp138–39). Talk with your doctor and get as much advice as possible. Remember, you can really make a difference by achieving gradual and sustained weight loss. The appropriate diet, when combined with regular exercise, will help you with this. See Chapter Six for dietary guidelines. Losing weight and then maintaining a new healthier weight can be difficult to do, which explains why so many people are overweight. Seek medical advice, particularly on the appropriate exercise. Also ask a dietitian for advice and join a weight-loss club to help motivate you.

Q How can I deal with the other risk factors for heart disease?

People with obesity are at increased risk of coronary artery disease, so it is vital to focus on all the risk factors. Stopping smoking (see pp151–52), doing regular exercise (see pp153–54), and of course eating healthily (see pp140–43) all help. As you lose weight, your lipid levels improve and your blood pressure comes down.

Q What about weight-loss medication?

If you have heart disease, you will need drugs to treat your heart symptoms and reduce your risk of further heart problems. If you are very overweight and have not succeeded in losing weight with a combination of diet and regular exercise, your doctor may consider a course of medication to help with weight loss. These drugs have side-effects and so your doctor will prescribe them only when they are really necessary.

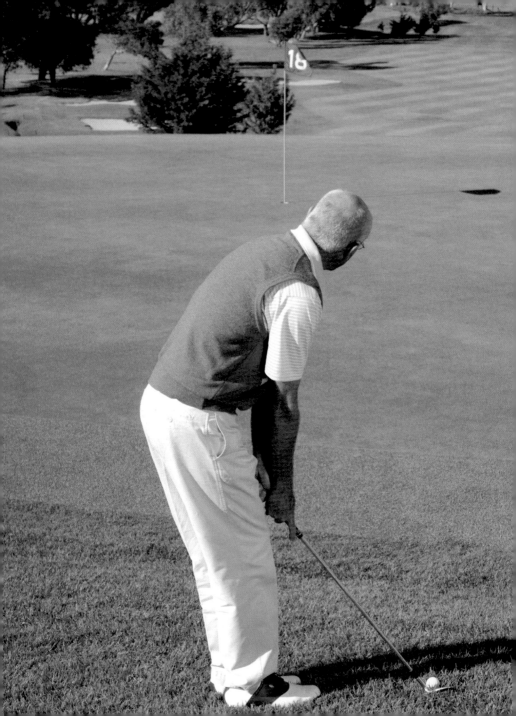

Long-term outlook

The understanding, diagnosis, and treatment of heart disease has advanced remarkably in the last few decades – in coronary artery disease, hypertension, and stroke (the three big killers) – and the outlook is much brighter today than it was in 1970. The near future appears bright as well – improved solutions are on the horizon.

Recurring problems

Q Do all heart problems recur at some time or other?

Most illnesses that comprise heart disease are chronic. However, coronary artery disease can be treated with the drugs that are now available and high blood pressure can be controlled.

Q Once treated, can the symptoms of heart failure recur?

Yes. Previously, you probably went to your doctor with shortness of breath on exertion, and tests revealed your heart was enlarged. You were probably treated with diuretics, an ACE inhibitor, and a beta-blocker. In the years ahead you may become breathless again and develop swollen ankles. Adjustments to your medication are usually effective but you may need additional treatment, like a pacemaker.

Q Why do I have to continue to take my blood pressure pills?

Because they keep your blood pressure stable. Most blood pressure pills work for 24 hours or less, after which time they will have been excreted from the body. High blood pressure is chronic – you simply have to take the pills regularly and forever.

Q Will my angina chest pain stay away once it is treated?

Yes and no. Angina is caused by an inadequate blood supply to the heart muscle cells. Most surgical treatments, including angioplasty, work by increasing the supply of blood, and most nonsurgical treatments lower the demand of the heart cells. However, the atherosclerosis in the coronary arteries continues, so further narrowing and chest pain may occur in the future. Nitroglycerine (see p108) can resolve an episode of chest pain, but further treatment may be necessary.

Complications

Q Can some anti-arrhythmia drugs cause a more serious arrhythmia?

Yes, but only rarely if they are properly monitored. One serious arrhythmia is a form of ventricular tachycardia (see p64), where the heart rate beats between 200–250 per minute. The ECG of the heart has a distinct pattern known as *torsades de pointes* (French for "twisting the points"). Many drugs and classes of drug that are used to abolish (or prevent) arrhythmias can cause *torsades de pointes* to occur. It is more likely to develop if your heart rate is slow or you have a low level of potassium in the blood (a frequent result of taking diuretics).

Q Can cardiac treatments cause allergic responses?

Yes, occasionally. Sometimes the agent that triggers the allergic reaction can be the dye used in X-ray imaging (cardiac catheterization) or it may simply be a cardiac medication. The allergy may not just cause a rash that can be treated with an antihistamine and then goes away. It may involve a serious body-wide response that leads to wheezing and a drop in blood pressure.

Q Can my doctor "overshoot" when treating my high blood pressure?

Yes, it's possible and when it occurs, a patient tends to feel tired, lethargic, and dizzy. The correct approach is to add one medication at a time so that blood pressure ideally falls 10/5 with each medication adjustment. Doctors should not increase an old or add a new medication more rapidly than once per week. The reduction in blood pressure is then slow and typically does not produce unwanted symptoms. However, even if these rules are followed, a particular patient may respond with an exaggerated drop in blood pressure.

Q Are there any complications from bypass surgery?

There may be several. Some people undergoing CABG (see pp100–101) may experience a myocardial infarction or stroke in the days after surgery. People with pre-existing lung disease have compromised breathing, while others may develop major wound infections or have a stroke. Arrhythmias, such as atrial fibrillation, are quite common, but the heart usually returns to a normal rhythm within a day or two. Sometimes a slow heart rate means a pacemaker is needed.

Q My doctor has prescribed statins to help lower my cholesterol. Are statins risk-free?

No. Statins are known to interfere with blood tests that measure liver function. Typically, these changes are minimal, reversible when the statins are stopped, and are rarely accompanied by signs of disease. So statins can be continued as long as liver function blood tests remain stable. However, another side-effect is muscle aching, which can progress to muscle destruction – this can be a reason to discontinue statins.

Q Is long-term anti-coagulation too risky?

People take anti-coagulation drugs such as warfarin in the long term following a mechanical valve replacement (see p120) or a thromboembolic event such as a blood clot (see p59). People with atrial fibrillation (see p63) may also need to take it permanently. However, dosage of oral warfarin can be problematic: too high leads to the risk of bleeding; too low can lead to a recurrence of blood clots. Even though the level should be checked frequently, it is difficult to be consistent in the therapeutic range. Nevertheless, it has been proven absolutely that the relative risk of maintaining long-term anti-coagulation treatment is far less than the risk of no anti-coagulation at all.

Q I've had a pacemaker inserted. Will there be any complications?

Although complications are very unlikely, pacemakers can cause soreness and very occasionally may cause an infection, in which case they need to be removed. The wires that link the pacemaker to the heart usually settle down within 48 hours or so. People who have had a pacemaker inserted can damage it in a fall or an accident, but this is rare. If you think you have done so you should contact your doctor at once. Sometimes, wear and tear brought on by everyday movement and activity may cause a malfunction. Again, contact your doctor if you think this has happened. Typically, the battery pack needs to be replaced every 10 years.

RISKS ASSOCIATED WITH A HEART TRANSPLANT

Recipients of a heart transplant will have failed to respond to traditional heart therapy. They are carefully screened for co-existing illness (cancer, diabetes, peripheral vascular disease, etc.) and probably would not survive for more than a few weeks without a transplant. Nearly 70 per cent of heart-transplant recipients are alive five years after the transplant and 50 per cent ten years after.

The risks of a heart transplant are:

DEATH Associated with the operation (10–15 per cent).

REJECTION The donor heart is a foreign substance and will be attacked by the recipient's immune system.

INFECTION Immunosuppressive drugs prevent rejection of the new heart, but make the recipient prone to infection.

MALIGNANCY The immunosuppressive drugs regime makes the heart recipient more vulnerable to cancer.

KIDNEY FAILURE Immunosuppressive drugs can be toxic to the kidneys, causing them to fail.

GRAFT CORONARY ARTERY DISEASE The transplanted heart develops coronary atherosclerosis (see p56). This can set in very early, suddenly, and then progress at an alarming rate.

Q Medications have side-effects, so should I really be taking something indefinitely?

Despite real benefits – sometimes they save lives and frequently they improve quality of life – all medications have potential side-effects. There is no way, however, to anticipate very rare side-effects until they present themselves, perhaps years after a drug is approved and on the market. That said, it's important to realize that the vast majority of people do not experience side-effects from their medications. Your doctor will weigh the potential benefits with the possible risks of each medication in order to develop an appropriate regimen for your condition. Since a significant number of cardiovascular medicines are prescribed in order to prolong life as well as minimize cardiac symptoms, it is crucial to take them as prescribed.

Q How can I know if my medication is causing a side-effect?

You may not know. If you suspect that you have developed a reaction to a medication, contact your doctor to discuss your symptoms. Don't stop taking the medication on your own. Some cardiac medications, such as beta-blockers, must be discontinued gradually. Before starting any new medication, discuss the possible side-effects with your doctor. Explain about other medicines you're taking, including nutritional supplements and vitamins, since interactions can also cause side-effects. Some side-effects are only identified by blood tests.

Q Do I have to take these medications forever?

Possibly. Many cardiovascular disorders are chronic illnesses that at present have no cure, so medications to treat these conditions need to be taken indefinitely. The need for chronic medication will not change until treatments or therapies are developed that cure the underlying cardiovascular diseases.

Future treatments

Q How has treatment for a heart attack progressed in the last 50 years?

The treatment for a heart attack has progressed from simple bed rest to the administration of life-saving medications and catheter-based procedures that not only minimize the size of a heart attack, but in the best-case scenario can entirely abort the heart attack. Arrhythmias are recognised with modern monitoring equipment.

Q Can we expect similar advances in the future?

Yes, there's every chance. The cumulative results of medical, surgical, and catheter-based treatments in the last 30 years have resulted in substantial improvements in life expectancy and quality of life for most people with coronary artery disease. There is still a need for progress and innovation for therapies across the whole spectrum of coronary artery disease. The ultimate goal remains the prevention of atherosclerosis and cardiac disease altogether. However, when structural heart damage is unavoidable, we can expect treatments to be more effective and durable, and to involve less major surgery.

Q Is there a new therapy for treating damage to heart muscle following a heart attack?

Potentially, yes. One active area of research is focusing on stimulating the body's ability to generate new tiny blood vessels, which can restore blood flow to areas that have been depleted by blocked arteries. This process is called neovascularization, and can be looked upon as the body's own way of creating natural bypasses. Cardiac research is looking at various ways of encouraging this to happen through the use of chemicals, known as growth factors, and possibly by employing stem cells that can be derived from bone marrow.

Q Will valve repair always require a surgical procedure?

Not necessarily. Although standard surgical valve repair has dramatically improved over the past three decades, additional innovations are currently being explored. They have yet to be evaluated in rigorous studies and trials, but some have been enthusiastically adopted by surgeons. Novel catheter devices are also being evaluated in human trials to determine whether certain valve disorders may be treatable via catheters rather than necessitating surgical repair.

Q Are there therapies for heart failure on the horizon?

Yes, potentially. The ultimate therapeutic goals for heart failure (see pp71–75), which is the final common pathway for most cardiac diseases, is to regenerate or repair damaged heart muscle. One regeneration approach is gene therapy, which involves isolating specific cardiac genes – for instance, the gene that regulates the strength of heart muscle contraction – and administering them into heart muscle by various techniques. Another new approach involves using stem cells from a patient's bone marrow to determine whether they can generate new heart muscle cells.

Q Are any new devices being developed?

Yes. The need for improved interventions and options for people with advanced heart failure drives active research to develop novel mechanical heart pumps, such as new left ventricular assist devices (LVADs). Research is focusing on creating miniaturized pumps that are more durable and reliable. At present these long-term assist devices are fairly large, and require open-heart surgery to implant. A new generation of "micro-devices" is in development, with the ultimate goal of implanting the pumps via catheters alone.

Q Can established therapies be improved in the future?

Almost certainly. Not every research study of future therapies involves novel drugs or devices. Even now routine surgical procedure, such as bypass surgery, is being studied in large clinical trials to determine whether certain groups, such as those with coronary artery disease and a weakened heart muscle, derive benefit from the operation. Within the next few years, the crucial question as to whether bypass surgery is effective in this large group of patients may finally be resolved. In addition, in the near future large clinical trials will evaluate the use of standard valve surgeries and newer techniques in patients who have been diagnosed with moderate and severe mitral valve regurgitation (see p67).

Q If I have the chance, should I agree to participate in a clinical trial?

This is something that only you can decide. On the one hand, you may want the most cutting-edge intervention for your condition, or your doctor might have told you that there are no further conventional options available despite ongoing symptoms or disease progression. On the other hand, you may prefer to be treated only with those therapies that have a long, well-defined track record. Always discuss potential participation in a clinical trial with your doctor. If you agree to participate, you have to sign an informed consent form, which means you are fully aware of what is involved.

Q If I sign up to participate in a clinical trial can I change my mind?

Yes. You can change your mind at any point. Even after you sign an informed consent form, you remain free to change your mind and not to participate in a clinical trial. You can even leave a trial for whatever reason, without forfeiting access to other standard treatment.

Useful addresses

British Heart Foundation
14 Fitzhardinge Street, London W1H 6DH
Tel: 020 7935 0185
Website: www.bhf.org.uk

Heart UK
7 North Road, Maidenhead, Berkshire SL6 1PE
Tel: 0845 450 5988
Email: ask@heartuk.org.uk
Website: www.heartuk.org.uk

The British Cardiac Patients Association
2 Station Road, Swavesey,
Cambridge CB24 5QJ
Tel: 01954 202022
Email: Enquiries@BCPA.co.uk
Website: www.bcpa.co.uk

Children's Heart Association
26 Elizabeth Drive, Helmshore
Rossendale, Lancashire BB4 4JB
Tel: 01706 221988
Email: information@heartchild.info
Website: www.heartchild.info

Heart Research UK
Suite 12D, Joseph's Well, Leeds LS3 1AB
Tel: 0113 234 7474
Email: info@heartresearch.org,uk
Website: www.heartresearch.org.uk

Blood Pressure Association
60 Cranmer Terrace, London SW17 0QS
Tel: 020 8772 4994
Website: www.bpassoc.org.uk

Chest, Heart & Stroke Scotland
65 North Castle Street, Edinburgh EH2 3LT
Tel: 0131 225 6963
Email: admin@chss.org.uk
Website: www.chss.org.uk

Irish Heart Foundation
4 Clyde Road, Ballsbridge, Dublin 4
Tel: 0353 1 6685001
Website: www.irishheart.ie

Northern Ireland Chest, Heart and Stroke Association
21 Dublin Road, Belfast BT2 7HB
Tel: 028 9032 0184
Website: www.nichsa.com

QUIT
211 Old Street, London EC1V 9NR
Tel: 020 7251 1551
Email: info@quit.org.uk
Website: www.quit.org.uk

Diabetes UK Central Office
Macleod House, 10 Parkway
London NW1 7AA
Tel: 020 7424 1000
Email: info@diabetes.org.uk
Website: www.diabetes.org.uk

National Health Service
www.nhsdirect.nhs.uk
Tel: 0845 4647

Index

A

ACE inhibitors 97, 105, 106, 116,
117, 129, 176
age 102, 136
heart problems in old age 34, 62,
65, 66, 71, 164–5
menopause in women 26, 34, 169,
170
AICD (automatic implanted
caradioverter defibrillator) 116
alcohol consumption 47, 48, 73, 75,
145, 147, 148, 158
alpha-blockers 105, 107
angina 54–5, 68, 89, 176
and diabetes 109, 171
and lifestyle 131, 147, 153, 155,
157
recurrence danger 40
treatment 82, 108–9, 155, 157, 176
in women 168, 170
angiography 74, 87, 88–9, 99, 176
angioplasty and stent treatment 70,
88, 89, 97, 98–9, 121, 165, 172
angiotensin II receptor antagonists
105, 106, 115, 116, 117
anticoagulants 66, 98, 113, 119, 120,
121, 178
aorta 13, 15, 18, 23, 30, 31, 101
arrhythmias 60–6, 164
and AICD 64, 66, 95, 116
and cocaine 48, 49
and pregnancy 170
treatment of 66, 84, 94, 95, 110–13,
116, 177
arteries 11, 13-16, 18, 21, 23–25,
30–1, 34
narrowing 37, 51, 54, 56–7, 59, 87,
176, 179
arterioles 11, 24, 54
arteriosclerotic cardiovascular disease 102
aspirin 95, 97, 129, 172
atheromata 38, 51, 151
atherosclerosis 37, 51, 54, 56–7, 59,
87, 176, 179
atrial
fibrillation 47, 61, 63, 65, 66, 67,
110, 112, 113, 178
premature contraction (APC) 61, 63, 66
septal defect 166
systole 19, 21
atrioventricular (AV) block 60, 66
atrioventricular nodes 20–1, 27–8, 83
atrium 14, 15, 17, 19, 20, 21, 27, 30–1

B

bacteria 37, 59, 76–7
beta-blockers 97, 105, 107–13, 129,
176, 180
and arrhythmias 110, 111, 112, 113
blood clots 44, 55, 56, 58, 59, 95,
113, 153
anticoagulants *see* anticoagulants

deep vein thrombosis (DVT) 169, 170
blood pressure 17, 22–3, 25
  and age 25, 34, 36, 86, 106, 164–5
  changes 36–7
  diastolic and systolic 22, 25, 36, 80,
    96
  ethnicity and family history 35
  high *see* high blood pressure
  low 37
  management of 24, 94
  measurement 22, 80–1
  optimum 36
blood tests 90–1
BMI (body mass index) 136–7, 173
breathlessness 58, 67, 96, 115, 116, 176
bypass surgery 89, 97, 98, 101, 172,
  178, 182, 183

C

C Reactive Protein (CRP) 39, 50, 91
caffeine 40, 63-4
calcium channel blockers 105, 107–13
cardiac catheter 23, 74, 77, 87, 88–9,
  98, 167, 177, 181, 182
cardiac markers 91
cardiomyopathy 51, 73, 96, 147, 167
cardiopulmonary resuscitation (CPR)
  18, 95
cardiopulmonary stress tests 74, 85
cardiovascular disease 11, 13, 36, 85
  and allergies 177
  blood tests 90
  and ethnicity 35

  and lifestyle 40–5, 47–8, 50–1, 90, 146
  repeat, danger of 40
  and statins 103
  see also individual conditions
chest pain, causes of 58, 70, 73, 87,
  89, 91, 108, 154
children 60, 63, 166–7
  see also pregnancy
cholesterol
  absorption prevention 103
  and age 34, 102
  blood tests 90
  diet to lower 126, 132, 133, 147,
    148–9, 172
  and family history 35
  and fat intake 142, 144, 149
  HDL 38–9, 51, 90, 104, 144, 148, 153
  LDL 38–9, 50, 51, 90, 102, 103,
    104, 142, 144, 148
  levels after heart attack 129
  and lifestyle 41, 50, 102, 148, 153
  medication to lower 102–4, 129,
    148, 178
  total serum 103
  triglyceride levels 148, 172
chordae tendinae 15, 118
circulatory system 10–13, 29–31,
  44–5, 107, 109, 111, 116
clinical trials 183
congenital heart disease 67, 68, 70,
  77, 85, 87, 167, 169
coronary artery bypass graft (CABG)
  97, 101, 116, 165, 178, 183
coronary artery disease 54–5, 57, 89
  and cholesterol *see* cholesterol

and cocaine 49
and diabetes 171, 172
and ethnicity 35
and heart failure 73, 74
and lifestyle 44–5, 47, 48, 132–3,
    147, 151, 153, 165, 173
rehabilitation programmes 100,
    124–9, 131, 153–4, 157
and stress 158
treatment of 58, 95, 97–101, 108,
    164, 165, 172, 176
in women 168, 170
creatine kinase (CK) 91
CT scans 74, 89

D

DC cardioversion 64, 95, 112, 113
deep vein thrombosis (DVT) 169, 170
defibrillators, implantable 64, 66, 95,
    110, 112, 113, 116
depression 42, 126, 130, 159, 160–1
diabetes
    and heart problems 40–1, 51, 90,
        102, 106, 107, 109, 111, 171-2
    and lifestyle 147, 153, 165, 172
diet
    and alcohol *see* alcohol
    cholesterol-lowering 126, 132, 133,
        148–9
    fat intake 142, 143, 144, 147, 149
    heart-healthy 133, 140–5, 147, 149,
        158, 173
    salt intake, limiting 75, 143, 150

and stress 158
and water intake, importance of
    143, 158
weight-loss 126, 127, 132, 133, 147,
    173
    see also exercise; weight
digitalis 112, 113
diuretics 96, 105, 106, 115, 117, 118,
    176, 177
    see also fluid retention
dizziness 36, 73, 165, 177
driving 126, 131
drugs
    medication *see* medication
    recreational 48–9, 73, 96
ductus arteriosus 30, 31, 166, 167

E

ECG test 65, 82-4, 91, 129, 166
echocardiography 67, 74, 77, 82,
    84–5, 121, 129, 166
emotional support 126, 127, 133
endocarditis 59, 76–7, 96
ethnicity 35
exercise
    and age 165
    cardiac rehabilitation programme
        100, 124–7, 129, 153, 158
    recommended levels of 40–1, 75,
        132, 153, 154, 155
    and sex 156, 157
    and stress 133, 158
    see also diet

F

family history 35, 73
fatigue 70, 73, 76, 116, 177
fibrates 103, 104
fluid retention 67, 70, 73, 75, 115
   see also diuretics
future treatments 181–3

G

gender 34, 35, 36, 41, 86
   see also women
gene therapy 35, 182

H

heart attack
   causes 37, 58, 59, 91, 96
   and cocaine 48–9
   and CRP blood test 90
   and depression 160
   and diabetes 51
   and ECG 84
   and exercise 153
   and family history 35
   gene 35
   recovery 124–7, 129–31
   recurrence danger 40, 108
   and rehabilitation programmes 100,
      124–7, 129, 153, 158
   and sex 156, 157
   treatment 58, 94, 129–30, 181
   in women 170

heart failure
   abdominal symptoms 74
   and age 34, 164
   and alcohol consumption 145
   causes of 71–2, 73–5, 111, 115
   in children 167
   congestive 37, 47, 68, 73
   and ethnicity and family history 35, 73
   treatment 75, 115–17, 182
   and viruses 75
heart murmurs, in children 166
heart muscle 19, 21, 27–8
   damage 57, 67, 71, 72, 74–5, 94,
      181, 182
heart scans 74
heart size 14, 29
heart transplant 89, 116, 167, 179
high blood pressure
   and age 164, 165
   and contraceptive pill 169
   definition of 80–1
   and diabetes 171
   and gender 86
   and heart failure 115, 117
   and lifestyle 36, 37, 41, 47, 49, 50,
      150, 151, 153, 165
   "overshooting" 177
   and pregnancy 106, 169, 170
   and retinal blood vessels 37, 96
   and stress 44, 133
   and strokes 36
   treatment 85, 96, 105–7, 165, 172,
      176, 177
   see also blood pressure
homocysteine 39, 90

HRT 168
hypertrophy 72, 164

I, K

infective endocarditis 67, 76, 118, 167
inotropics 96, 115
intravascular sonography 89
ischemic heart disease 59, 85
kidney disease 37, 44, 105, 164, 179

L

left ventricular assist device (LVAD)
    116, 182
lifestyle *see* alcohol; diet; exercise;
    smoking
lipid levels 127, 173

M, N

medication
    risks of side-effects 180
    tips for taking and understanding 130
    see also individual conditions
menopause 26, 34, 168, 169, 170
mitral valve 15, 16, 21, 70
    prolapse 77
    regurgitation 67, 118, 183
    replacement 119
    stenosis 67, 118–19
MRA scan 89

MRI scans 74
myocardial infarction *see* heart attack
neovascularization 181
nitroglycerine (NTG) 96, 108, 176

O

obesity 40–1, 90
    childhood 51
    incidence of 50
    and weight-loss 50, 126, 127, 132,
        133, 147, 173
open-heart surgery 119, 182
oxygen supply to heart 28, 30, 45, 47,
    48, 72, 94

P

pacemakers, implantable 64, 66, 95,
    110, 112, 113, 116, 179
palpitations 61, 63, 113, 170
    see also arrhythmias
peripheral arterial disease 90
peripheral vascular disease 37, 44, 51,
    171
personality type 42
platelets 56, 76, 95
Plavix 129
pregnancy
    and BMI 136
    heart development in the womb
        29–31
    and heart failure 73, 117

and high blood pressure 106, 169, 170

and infant heart problems 166

see also children; women

pulmonary

oedema 96

regurgitation 70, 118

stenosis 118

valves 14, 15, 69, 70

veins 13, 14, 21, 72

pump, heart as 10, 12, 14, 17, 18–23, 29, 30

R

red wine 46

rehabilitation programmes 100, 124–7, 129, 153, 158

reperfusion 94, 95

resins 103, 104

respiratory disease 107, 109, 111

rheumatic heart disease 67, 68, 70, 119

S

sex and relationships 156, 157

shift work 43

sick sinus syndrome 61, 112

smoking 41, 44–5, 90, 125, 165

and contraceptive pill 169

passive 45

stopping 47, 126–7, 132–3, 151–2, 173

and stress 42, 158

statins 97, 102–3, 104, 178

stem cells 182

stent treatment 70, 88, 89, 97, 98–9, 121, 165, 172

stress levels 41, 42–3, 131, 145

coping with 44, 126, 133, 158–9

strokes 35, 40, 47, 51, 90, 153, 164, 178

supraventricular tachycardia (SVT) 63, 113

sweating 55, 58

T

tachycardia 49, 63, 110, 113

ventricular 64, 66, 95, 113, 177

tricuspid valves 14, 15, 16, 17, 21, 70, 118

triglycerides 103, 104

troponins 91

V

vagus nerve 19

valves

aortic 15, 21, 68, 70, 118, 120, 164

artificial 77, 119–20, 121, 178

calcification 68

construction 16

disorders, treatment 118–21

mitral *see* mitral valves

pulmonary 14, 15, 69, 70, 118

repair, future treatments 182
replacement 70, 96, 119, 120–1, 178
St. Jude 119, 121
Starr-Edwards ball cage 119
stenosis 69, 70, 118–19, 166
surgery 116, 182, 183
tricuspid 14, 15, 16, 17, 21, 70, 118
vasodilators 105
veins 11–16, 21, 72
   leg, in bypass operations 101
vena cava 15, 21, 30, 31
ventricle 14–17, 19–22, 27–8
ventricular
   arrhythmias 64, 66, 95, 110
   hypertrophy 164
   premature contractions (VPC) 63,
      66, 113
   septal defect 166, 167
   systole 19, 21
   tachycardia (VT) 64, 66, 95, 113,
      177
Viagra 156
virus 73, 167

and contraceptive pill 169
and deep vein thrombosis (DVT)
   169
and diabetes 171
heart problems in 26, 169–70
and HRT 168, 170
and menopause 26, 34, 168, 169,
   170
see also pregnancy
work return 126, 131

W

warfarin 178
weight
   assessment of healthy 134–5
   and BMI (body mass index) 136–7,
      173
   and body shape 134–5, 136, 138–9
   see also diet
women

About the Authors

Robert Ascheim, MD, is a general
cardiologist specializing in coronary
artery disease and congestive heart
failure, and is an Associate Professor of
Medicine at Cornell University–Weill
Medical College, New York.
Deborah V. Davis Ascheim, MD, is
a cardiologist specializing in heart
disease and congestive heart failure.
She is Assistant Professor of Medicine
at Columbia University's College
of Physicians and Surgeons, and
head of the clinical trials group of
the International Center for Health
Outcomes and Innovation Research,
Mailman School of Public Health,
Columbia University.

About Dr Chris Davidson

Dr Davidson is a Senior Cardiologist
with the Brighton and Sussex University
Hospitals Trust and is Secretary-General
and Vice-President of the European
Federation of Internal Medicine.

For the publishers

Dorling Kindersley would like to thank:
Dr Penny Preston for her contribution
to the text of Chapters 6 & 7; Jo Walton
for picture research; Andi Sisodia for
proofreading; Margaret McCormack
for the index; Laura Palosuo for
additional editorial assistance;
and Vicky Read for additional
design assistance.

Picture credits

The publisher would like to thank the following for their kind permission to reproduce their photographs: (Key: a-above; b-below/bottom; c-centre; l-left; r-right; t-top)

7 Corbis: Andrew Brookes (r). Getty I2 PunchStock: Polka Dot. 6 Alamy Images: foodfolio (bc). jupiterimages: Fancy/HBSS (bl). PunchStock: Purestock (br). 7 Corbis: LWA-Dann Tardif (tr). jupiterimages: Asia Images (tl). PunchStock: Brand X Pictures (tc). 8-9 PunchStock: Brand X Pictures. 26 PunchStock: BananaStock. 32-33 jupiterimages: foodpix. 37 Science Photo Library: Paul Parker. 46 Getty Images: Maren Caruso. 52-53 Alamy Images: Phototake Inc.. 62 PunchStock: Fancy. 69 Science Photo Library: (b). 72 Science Photo Library. 78-79 PunchStock: Brand X Pictures. 84 Science Photo Library: Chris Gallagher. 86 Corbis: A. Inden/zefa. 88 Science Photo Library: (b). 92-93 Corbis: Rick Gomez. 112 Science Photo Library: AJ Photo. 114 jupiterimages: Fancy/HBSS. 127 Corbis: Hughes Martin. 128 jupiterimages. 133 PunchStock: Digital Vision. 155 Alamy Images: allOver photography. 156

PunchStock: Corbis. 159 PunchStock: BananaStock. 162-163 PunchStock: Comstock Images. 168 jupiterimages: Macduff Everton. 174-175 PunchStock: Fancy

Jacket images: Front: Corbis: Roulier/Turiot/photocuisine bl; Getty Images: Jens Haas br; David Madison bc. Back: Corbis: Marianna Day Massey/ZUMA tl; Getty Images: Peter Dazeley tc; Shinya Sasaki/NEOVISION tr

All other images © Dorling Kindersley
For further information see: www.dkimages.com